OBESITY

OBESITY

The Biography

Sander L. Gilman

OXFORD

OBESITY

The Biography

Sander L. Gilman

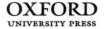

OXFORD
UNIVERSITY PRESS

OXFORD

UNIVERSITY PRESS

Great Clarendon Street, Oxford OX2 6DP

Oxford University Press is a department of the University of Oxford.
It furthers the University's objective of excellence in research, scholarship,
and education by publishing worldwide in

Oxford New York

Auckland Cape Town Dar es Salaam Hong Kong Karachi
Kuala Lumpur Madrid Melbourne Mexico City Nairobi
New Delhi Shanghai Taipei Toronto

With offices in

Argentina Austria Brazil Chile Czech Republic France Greece
Guatemala Hungary Italy Japan Poland Portugal Singapore
South Korea Switzerland Thailand Turkey Ukraine Vietnam

Oxford is a registered trade mark of Oxford University Press
in the UK and in certain other countries

Published in the United States
by Oxford University Press Inc., New York

© Sander L. Gilman 2010

The moral rights of the author have been asserted
Database right Oxford University Press (maker)

First published 2010

British Library Cataloguing in Publication Data

Data available

Library of Congress Cataloging in Publication Data

Library of Congress Control Number: 2010923435

Typeset by SPI Publisher Services, Pondicherry, India
Printed in Great Britain
on acid-free paper by
Clays Ltd., St Ives Plc

ISBN 978-0-19-955797-4

1 3 5 7 9 10 8 6 4 2

CONTENTS

List of illustrations   vi
Prologue   ix

1   The exemplary patient   1

2   Obesity from the Ancients to the beginning
of the Modern Age   21

3   Obesity from the Renaissance to
the Enlightenment   38

4   The battle between science and morality for
the cure of obesity   58

5   A somatic *or* a psychological treatment of
obesity   80

6   New causes; new solutions for obesity   113

7   The "Orient" battles obesity   130

8   Globesity and the Public's health   158

Glossary   173
Notes   177
Further reading   203
Index   207

LIST OF ILLUSTRATIONS

1. Daniel Lambert, "A Very Large Man"   2
2. "Phiz" [Hablot Knight Browne], "The Fat Boy Awake on This Occasion Only"   6
3. "Phiz" [Hablot Knight Browne], "Mary and the Fat Boy"   10
4. Hippocrates   22
5. A. Cornelius Celsus   26
6. Galen   27
7. Luigi Cornaro   39
8. George Cheyne   53
9. A large gentleman with a walking stick   60
10. Samuel Johnson   62
11. Carl von Noorden   82
12. Edmund Bristow, "Dispensing of Medical Electricity"   88
13. Sir William Withey Gull   95
14. A man, aged 37, suffering from infantilism (Type Brissaud) and a physical degenerative disorder—possibly thyroid   99
15. Eadweard Muybridge, "A Gargantuan Woman Walking"   108

16. An earnest discussion of dietetic methods
    of achieving longevity during the Ming period
    (1368–1644)   133

17. James Gillray, "A Voluptary under
    the Horrors of Digestion"   163

18. A female Hottentot   167

PROLOGUE

PROLOGUE

We are, according to most public health authorities, in the midst of a pandemic of "globesity," (global obesity) a term coined in 2001 by the World Health Organization. But is globesity a disease itself or is it a symptom of underlying physiological or psychological illnesses, or a sign of social excess and thus not a disease in the medical sense at all? And is it really new? Given the predicted impact of obesity in the twenty-first century on personal health as well as its social and economic costs for the global economy, the biography of obesity, unlike other medical categories, may well be a necessity in determining our medical as well as social responses to this ancient concern.

This volume is appearing in a series of volumes on the "biography of diseases." Obesity is not itself a disease but rather a phenomenological category that reflects the visible manifestation of body size, which potentially can have multiple (as well as multifactorial) causes. No one dies from obesity. One dies from those pathologies that may result from extreme overweight. Indeed, obesity may only be a tertiary cause of morbidity or mortality: it may lead to diabetes, which may lead to vascular disease. Or, and here is the rub, it may not. Many people have and do live with excess weight but the notion of being healthy and overweight seems impossible to imagine in our day. If you are fat, you are sick. Every medical system we shall examine has the category of obesity as a state of ill health.

What is important is that the boundaries between the obese and, therefore, unhealthy body and the stout, plump, heavy, well-fleshed, stately, but healthy body are constantly shifting. What is a corpulent but healthy body in one system can and does easily become an obese and ill one in the next. The boundary between acceptable and unacceptable weight and body size is always determined within the medical system and within the general culture. Medicine is a part of general culture and the general culture is shaped by medicine. Today we have drawn the line that delineates obesity just as clearly as it has been drawn in the past, but in a different place. And we now define it as a major public health dilemma much as we have defined tuberculosis or leprosy in the past.

Moreover, our present image of an epidemic of obesity relies on the model of infectious disease and demands a single, clearly defined cause for this disease, much as has been done with other recent epidemics of infectious diseases from tuberculosis to swine flu. The bacteriologist Robert Koch's postulates concerning the nature of infectious disease, developed in the 1890s, demanded that there be an absolute relationship shown between the specific cause of an infection and its appearance in an animal. Obesity is not a disease within the same model (although as we shall see that there is an ongoing desire that at least some obesity may well be the result of viral infection and, therefore, fit Koch's postulates.)

The modern model of obesity has its roots, however, much more in the extrapolation of mortality and morbidity from an epidemiological model of disease. In 1942 Louis Dublin (1882–1969), a statistician and epidemiologist with the Metropolitan Life Company (MetLife), examined the association between mortality and weight among the four million people insured by his company. He classified people based on height, weight, and body frame (small, medium, or large). He was interested in the use of statistics to quantify the occurrence of diseases, thinking that knowing risk would help to increase people's life expectancy by changing their actions. The individuals insured by MetLife who maintained the average weight for 25-year-olds seemed to have greater longevity than those who were outside the weight range. Based on these findings, he determined that people who maintained weight in an ideal range would live longer and be at lower risk for MetLife to insure. He published tables containing ideal weight for individuals based on their height and body frame.

The bias in this claim is clear: Dublin's population was heavily male, white, middle-class, and urban. But based on this population the "body mass index" (BMI) was developed, which seems to be a scientific model of healthy and ill bodies based on their weight and height. The BMI is a mathematical value calculated by weight in kilograms divided by height in meters squared (kg/m^2). It remains the prime indicator for the definition of obesity today and is highly correlated with health risk. Thus, today underweight is indicated by a BMI of less than 18.5; normal weight by a BMI of 18.5 to 24.9; overweight by a BMI of 25 to 29.9; and obesity by a BMI of 30 or greater. As BMI increases, so does the risk of morbidity and mortality. As we shall see in the chapter on China, scientists in Asia have contested the use of "Western" models of risk, such as the BMI standards, seeing them as inappropriate for understanding the health of Asian populations. But even Western scientists, while using BMI models, doubt their accuracy. The range has been altered downward over time to include more and more individuals in higher risk categories. Today a variety of alternatives to BMI have been proposed, including waist circumference measurement. Males with a waist circumference greater than 40 inches and females with a waist circumference greater than 35 inches are believed to be at an increased risk for a wide range of illnesses from type 2 diabetes to hypertension and cardiovascular disease. But all such body measures rely on the populations from which the standards have been extrapolated and the fact of the matter is that all of these populations are constantly in flux. While the risk factors for an ever-widening range of diseases are now seen to be correlated with weight, the population from which the standards of weight are taken may well have other predetermining factors for those diseases. This increased emphasis on higher weight as the source of an extensive range of costly illnesses has made obesity the new focus of public anxiety in the twenty-first century.

Obesity has today triggered a moral panic, much as did AIDS in the 1980s, with real political and social implications. It is also evident that the impact of being overweight on health is real and our medical responses are determined as much by the developments of medical knowledge and technology as by the social meaning associated with the disease. Constructing diseases such as obesity does not always mean inventing them. Often, real pathological experiences are rethought as part of a new pattern that can be then discerned, diagnosed, and treated. Obesity as a category has been the subject of such a public rethink over the past decades. It has become the target of public health campaigns and spurred a global reassessment of where the sources of danger for the general public may lie. Fat people certainly exist in the world, but the boundaries of what defines "fat" and the meanings attached to it are constantly shifting. Such a rethink mixes together and stirs many qualities, to provide a compelling story that defines obesity as the "new public health epidemic." This is not to discount the costs, both personal and national, that overweight can accrue, but to understand why, in the twenty-first century, we have suddenly seen the "moral panic," which was associated in the 1980s with HIV and AIDS as a potentially global disease, being transferred to obesity. Indeed, the moral panic about obesity seems to have filled a gap left by the restructuring of the moral panic about AIDS, today mistakenly seen as curable, just as AIDS filled the gap left in the West by the "conquest" of syphilis with the widespread introduction of antibiotics in the 1950s.

Moral panics can alter the meaning and impact of real situations in the world. The very term had its origin in Jock Young's study of the beginnings of the British drug scene.[1] It has since been used to analyse social "epidemics," such as child abuse and, of course, the American "war on drugs." No one would be foolhardy enough to claim that child abuse or drug addiction did not exist, but the moral panic associated with these categories over the past decades is the result of heightened anxiety about social instability. Obesity clearly exists in the world; but how it is defined is culturally, not scientifically, limited and its centrality in the mental universe of any given individual is heavily dependant on the role of anxiety associated with it. In our dieting culture, obesity has come to have meanings well beyond health and beauty; it has become a danger to the body politic because of the mounting costs of those diseases associated today with obesity. This very short biography of obesity will thus trace its history within medicine but always acknowledging that this history shapes and is shaped by the meanings attached to the obese body (however defined) in the general culture.

Obesity appears as a medical category of diagnosis in the most ancient medical texts available. Indeed, in the West there seems to be no medical system that did not and does not include obesity as either disease or symptom and no medical system that does not offer some type of intervention from dieting to exercise to psychological or moral treatment to "cure" obesity. What is labeled as globesity is, in fact, the most recent version of an obsession with bodily control in society and the promise of universal health through all forms of medicine. Its modern iteration, however, comes with an unstated and complex history. If, said the ancients, you would only eat well, sacrifice to the gods, avoid certain foods, undertake rigorous exercise, then your health would improve or simply never decline. Yet there have been changes in eating patterns and the concomitant meaning of body weight throughout history. Perhaps in the twenty-first century these changes speed around the world more quickly than in the past. But the notion of a world in decay due to the growth of girth carries with it odd and complex subtexts.

What are the central implications of globesity? Is it social? Globesity, according to a publication of the Pan American Health Organization in 2002, "places the blame not on individuals but on globalization and development, with poverty as an exacerbating factor."[2] Is obesity really determined by global economics or is it equally a medical problem that has its origin in our genes? Is obesity the result of an infectious disease or a manifestation of a weakness of will? Or is it a combination of all or some of these proposed etiologies? For a weakness of will could arguably be a tendency deriving from an individual's genetic make-up. But what if the answer lies not in our genes or in our bodies but in our social environment? In the eighteenth century, obesity was understood as a problem of the affluent; today the affluent are more likely to have a personal trainer and a healthy diet, and it is the poorer classes in the "First World" who are more likely to be overweight as it is argued that they live in urban areas remote from sources of "healthy food." Indeed "fast food," often defined as "bad food," is generally cheaper than organic food! Yet what about obesity among the rural poor in the "developing countries," whose diets seem to consist of only "natural and local" foods? Latin and South America are seen as places where obesity and illness are now rampant among the rural poor, while in China the rural poor are understood as undernourished and ill. (Chapter 7 examines in detail how Western models of famine and obesity become a part of a "Chinese" means of understanding the body in the course of the modernization of China during the twentieth century.) Is obesity to be cured by diet or surgery, by psychotherapy or economic improvement, by healthier "food choices" or social relocation, by an anti-viral drug or by the promised magic bullet: the pill that lets you eat and do what you wish and still remain slim, young, healthy, and beautiful? Or perhaps by a combination of all of these, depending on how you are, where you live, and how you earn your livelihood?

Obesity is dangerous to society as well as to the individual because it is now globalized: in complex ways obesity is now (as smoking was) a sign of the deleterious effect of the modern (read: the American) influence on the body. Indeed, the argument in the twenty-first century is that the gains among the elderly through changes in lifestyle over the past decades, such as the abandonment of smoking, will be swamped by the "disabilities among the young," grown huge and ill through the pernicious effects of food. We have to restore the healthy mind of youth and thus heal the unhealthy body of society. This is the goal of obesity treatments of all kinds in the twenty-first century. This short history of obesity, beginning with the ancient Greeks and continuing to the twenty-first century, shows the ongoing concern with this unhealthy social body.

I

THE EXEMPLARY PATIENT

Who would be the best patient to tell the story of our modern concern with the obese body? If obesity alters and changes its meanings as radically as we will see in the course of our short biography, we would have to have a patient who was exposed to a wide range of diagnoses based on a diverse (and often contradictory) set of models for the overweight and unhealthy body. He or she would need to be a patient whose life extends across much of the nineteenth, twentieth, and twenty-first centuries. There is such an object of study: not a live patient, but a literary one. The history of obesity and its variants can be read in the tale of our exemplary obese patient: Charles Dickens' character "Fat Joe" and his legacy.

How does the history of real live (and dead) fat men in the eighteenth and early nineteenth centuries, such as the most famous "fat man" of the eighteenth century, Daniel Lambert [1770–1809], lead to the creation of a literary character, who in turn becomes a diagnostic category in allopathic medicine from the nineteenth to the twenty-first century? Our biography of Fat Joe focuses all of the debates about obesity in the world

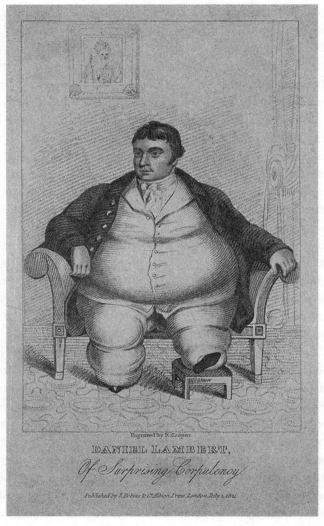

1. Daniel Lambert, "A Very Large Man." Stipple engraving by R. Cooper, 1821. (*Wellcome Collection*)

of medicine as it shaped a fictive character, who represented all of the overweight of his age and became a touchstone for discussions of obesity into the twenty-first century.

Daniel Lambert was the exemplary "real" obese man of the nineteenth century. By profession a jailer, Lambert came to represent the freakish nature of fat. George Meredith described London as "the Daniel Lambert of cities" and Herbert Spencer used the phrase "a Daniel Lambert of learning" A wax model of Lambert found its way to America and was shown in the Mix Museum in New Haven in 1813 and later in P. T. Barnum's famous American Museum. Lambert had been displayed as a wonder of nature along with giants and dwarfs much against his own desires. He was huge and yet the contemporary literature stressed that he neither drank nor ate "more than one dish at a meal" and after his death he was remembered as a man of great "temperance."[1] Other than his size, he was deemed to be of "perfect health: his breathing was free, his sleep undisturbed, and all of the functions of his body in excellent order."[2] In other words, he was huge but healthy and happy.

Lambert's early death (at the time he measured 5 ft. 1 in. in height and weighed 739 lb. (52 stones 11 lb.)) was bemoaned by fashionable London that had made him one of the sights that had to be visited when you were on the town. When he died, his body had to be removed from the room in which he was staying by demolishing a wall! As his body weight increased he went on a perpetual diet, without any decrease in his rate of weight gain. Lambert functions as an exemplar of a human being of great size, but he also acquires a social status that is attributable to his "freakish" body. Lambert was one of the "case studies" of obesity of the time that created much of the interest in obesity as part of the world of medical freakishness.

Indeed, Dr. T. Coe's earlier (1751) letter to the Royal Society about Mr. Edward Bright, the "fat man at Malden in Essex," has a certain breathless quality about it. Bright was "so extremely fat, and of such an uncommon bulk and weight, that I believe there to be very few, if any, such instances to be found in any country, or upon record in any books..."[3] According to Coe, Bright was descended from a lineage of "remarkably fat" people. Extremely fat as a child, he grew in size and weight over the years until at his death, at 30, he weighed more than 616 lb. (44 stones) at 5 ft. 9 in. He was "the gazing-stock and admiration of all people."[4] He ate "remarkably" and drank much beer, a gallon a day.[5] Those about him saw his "life as a burthen, and death as a happy release."[6] According to Coe, no respite could have been had by diet or therapy.

By 1872, the physician William Harvey stressed that the new scientific advances in "physiology and animal chemistry" had meant that one could treat obesity as a disease. Lambert became part of the medical literature, but in a very different tone. Harvey cited the case of Lambert, the fattest man on record at that time, and suggested that there seemed to have been no attempt to "arrest the progress of the disease" in Lambert's case.[7] More medical intervention, of the type available to nineteenth-century medicine, Harvey opined, could now have "cured" Lambert.

But it is in literature that the exemplary case for obesity is found. The character of Fat Joe in Charles Dickens' *Pickwick Papers* (1836) quickly became the touchstone for theories of obesity from those of endocrinologists to the psychoanalysts to contemporary geneticists. What indeed did Fat Joe suffer from and how does he become the classic eponym for obesity within modern medicine?

Dickens' interest in obesity is a fascination with the claim that the body's surface reveals its character. From our standpoint (and any viewer of the "Phiz" illustrations by Halbot K. Browne) everyone in *The Pickwick Papers* is fat. Yet Dickens presents two kinds of "fat": the first is Mr. Samuel Pickwick (and his middle-class friends) who is "fat-cheery" instead of "fat-bloated." Pickwick is plump and "charged with energy, solar or otherwise. He bursts, he beams, he bulges…His fatness…is scarcely even heavy." But the "fat-bloated" form of obesity seems to be incorporated in the servant, Joe, who is better known as "the fat boy."

He is regularly described as snoring "in a low and monotonous sound." Joe is comic because of his girth and what it implies:

> "Come along, Sir. Pray, come up," said the stout gentleman. "Joe!—damn that boy, he's gone to sleep again.—Joe, let down the steps." The fat boy rolled slowly off the box, let down the steps, and held the carriage door invitingly open. Mr. Snodgrass and Mr. Winkle came up at the moment. "Room for you all, gentlemen," said the stout man. "Two inside, and one out. Joe, make room for one of these gentlemen on the box. Now, Sir, come along," and the stout gentleman extended his arm, and pulled first Mr. Pickwick, and then Mr. Snodgrass, into the barouche by main force. Mr. Winkle mounted to the box, the fat boy waddled to the same perch, and fell fast asleep instantly.[8]

Sam Weller calls him "young dropsy,"[9] ironically seeing his sleepiness as a reflection of some unstated illness. Pickwick calls him a "young opium eater."[10] He is a freak, a body that "had never [been] seen in or out of a traveling convoy."[11] His is a truly obese body unlike that of the bourgeoisie characters. And it is seen as neither healthy nor "normal."

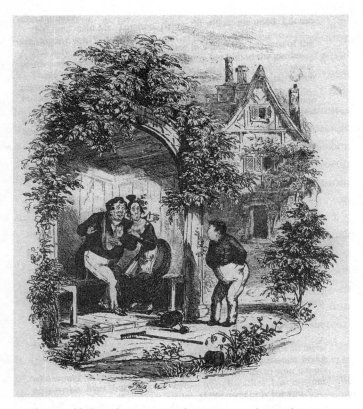

2. "Phiz" [Hablot Knight Browne], "The Fat Boy Awake on This Occasion Only," from Charles Dickens, *The Posthumous Papers of the Pickwick Club.* (*London: Chapman & Hall, 1836*)

There is one odd but effective moment very early in *The Pickwick Papers* where the question of Joe's obesity and his mental and emotional status is drawn into question. Joe accidentally observes an attempted seduction take place in the garden. Mr. Tracy Tupman is wooing the "spinster aunt"[12] Rachael Wardle, an odd match even in the world of Pickwick, for "young men, to spinster aunts, are as lighted gas to gunpowder."[13] Joe observes them and the seducer looks at Joe being "perfectly motionless, with his large circular eyes staring into the arbour, but without the slightest expression on his face that the most expert physiognomist could have referred to astonishment, curiosity, or any other known passion that agitates the human breast. Mr. Tupman gazed on the fat boy, and the fat boy stared at him; and the longer Mr. Tupman observed the utter vacancy of the fat boy's countenance, the more convinced he became that he either did not know, or did not understand, anything that had been going forward."[14]

But of course, Joe had understood all too well. As Tupman walks off "there was a sound behind them, as of an imperfectly suppressed chuckle. Mr. Tupman turned sharply round. No; it could not have been the fat boy; there was not a gleam of mirth, or anything but feeding in his whole visage." His fat physiognomy was unreadable but he knew what he had observed and turned it to his own advantage!

In Wilhelm Ebstein's late Victorian study of obesity, the first standard medical presentation of obesity as a physiological problem, the author quotes the eighteenth-century German essayist Georg Lichtenberg, who says that "there be people with such plump faces that they may laugh under their fat, so that the greatest physiognomist shall fail to notice it, while we poor slender creatures with our souls seated immediately beneath the epidermis, ever speak a language which can tell no lies."[15] Joe seems to be inscrutable in his obesity.

This is the reader's introduction to Joe at the very beginning of the novel. His stories may make the characters' flesh creep only because they seem not to be able to read his face. For Fat Boys' physiognomy seems not to mirror their character. And yet at the very conclusion of the novel, Dickens returns to the same scene in a different setting. He stumbles into another seduction, now undertaken by more individuals appropriate in terms of their ages, when he sees Mr. Augustus Snodgrass with his arm about his beloved Emily Wardle's waist:

"Wretched creature, what do you want here?" said the gentleman, who it is needless to say was Mr. Snodgrass.

To this the fat boy, considerably terrified, briefly responded, "Missis."

"What do you want me for," inquired Emily, turning her head aside, "you stupid creature?"

"Master and Mr. Pickwick is a-going to dine here at five," replied the fat boy.

"Leave the room!" said Mr. Snodgrass, glaring upon the bewildered youth.

"No, no, no," added Emily hastily. "Bella, dear, advise me."

Upon this, Emily and Mr. Snodgrass, and Arabella and Mary, crowded into a corner, and conversed earnestly in whispers for some minutes, during which the fat boy dozed.

"Joe," said Arabella, at length, looking round with a most bewitching smile, "how do you do, Joe?"

"Joe," said Emily, "you're a very good boy; I won't forget you, Joe."

"Joe," said Mr. Snodgrass, advancing to the astonished youth, and seizing his hand, "I didn't know you before. There's five shillings for you, Joe!"

"I'll owe you five, Joe," said Arabella, "for old acquaintance sake, you know;" and another most captivating smile was bestowed upon the corpulent intruder.

The fat boy's perception being slow, he looked rather puzzled at first to account for this sudden prepossession in his favour, and stared about him in a very alarming manner. At length his broad face began to show symptoms of a grin of proportionately broad dimensions; and then, thrusting half-a-crown into each of his pockets, and a hand and wrist after it, he burst into a horse laugh: being for the first and only time in his existence.

"He understands us, I see," said Arabella.

"He had better have something to eat, immediately," remarked Emily.[16]

Joe certainly understands. He understands the moment of seduction he has observed. He certainly understands the double sense of Arabella's statement that she will not forget him, a two-edged statement that has to do with monetary reward but also an acknowledgement of him as a human being. He may be "slow" but he clearly understands the sexual tension in the room and the power that that grants him. His physiognomy is completely readable by all. He smiles and he laughs, as for once he is in control of the situation, or is he?

And the company sends the servant Mary off with Joe to make sure that he does not again expose lovers to the forces of social control. It is the laughter (that had also signaled Joe's first sense of awareness in his observation of the earlier seduction) that makes them anxious. They immediately sit down to feed Joe's appetite. Mary's feeding of Joe is to draw his attention away from the desire shown by the lovers and Joe unexpectedly offers Mary some of the food with which she was bribing him:

The fat boy assisted Mary to a little, and himself to a great deal, and was just going to begin eating when he suddenly

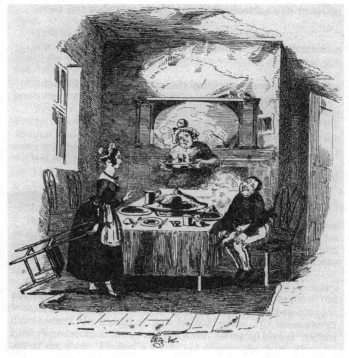

3. "Phiz," [Hablot Knight Browne], "Mary and the Fat Boy," from Charles Dickens, *The Posthumous Papers of the Pickwick Club*. (*London: Chapman & Hall, 1836*)

laid down his knife and fork, leaned forward in his chair, and letting his hands, with the knife and fork in them, fall on his knees, said, very slowly —

'I say! How nice you look!'

This was said in an admiring manner, and was, so far, gratifying; but still there was enough of the cannibal in the young gentleman's eyes to render the compliment a double one.

'Dear me, Joseph,' said Mary, affecting to blush, 'what do you mean?'

The fat boy, gradually recovering his former position, replied with a heavy sigh, and, remaining thoughtful for a few moments, drank a long draught of the porter. Having achieved this feat, he sighed again, and applied himself assiduously to the pie.[17]

The question of Joe's unexpected attraction to Mary startles the reader in Dickens' use of the image of the cannibal. He ironically has us see the Fat Boy reducing Mary from an object of erotic desire to one of gustatory pleasure. Yet the "heavy sigh" points to a very different desire. He knows what object of desire is available to him. Following this exchange, Joe returns to Pickwick with a note from Emile Wardle. He comments to Sam Weller about the servant girl Mary (in whom Weller is more than interested) that "'I say,' said Joe, who was unusually loquacious, 'what a pretty girl Mary is, isn't she? I am SO fond of her, I am!' Mr. Weller made no verbal remark in reply; but eyeing the fat boy for a moment, quite transfixed at his presumption, led him by the collar to the corner, and dismissed him with a harmless but ceremonious kick."[18] Even Fat Boys can show desire!

The Fat Boy quickly becomes a figure in the medical literature of Dickens' age. In 1859, the British colonial surgeon W. G. Don, reporting from India, presented the case of a twelve year old "Hindoo boy, known in the streets of Bombay under the soubriquet of the 'Fat Boy'."[19] The echo of Dickens in this colonial report is clear. Don's "Fat Boy" had become very fat at the age of two until, "His whole body is now encased in an immense mass of solid adipose tissue, which hangs in pendulous folds over his chest and hips, and the flexures of his limbs." At 12, he is 48½ inches tall weighing 206 lb. (14 stones 10 lb.). He seems in good health except for "a difficulty breathing" but his "appearance is extremely odd" as he "walks with difficulty, and when tired rests himself by leaning his pendulous abdomen against a wall." While he seems normally developed for a 12-year-old, "the genital organs, however, are not larger than those of an infant, while the testes are very small, and seem either to be undeveloped or to have become atrophied." He is, however, "highly intelligent."

Joe, however, became a medical case study of obesity against Dickens' much more complex image of obesity as yet one of the manifestations of human nature. It was read as an example of the obesity of youth. As Edward Jukes noted in 1833: "Fat, when moderately diffused over the body, indicates a sound state of health, and an easy disposition, gives a symmetry to the figure, and (which by many is valued more than all these) it contributes much to the beauty of the countenance; but on the contrary, where it accumulates to excess, it becomes an absolute disease, and is frequently the cause of death, particularly in habits where some chronic disorder has preceded it, or where acute attacks of disease have been aggravated by its presence."[20] The causes, according to Dickens' contemporary, are either "occasioned by indulging in the use of highly nutritious foods" or, as in the case of the Fat Boy, "a peculiarity of constitution predisposing to this state."[21] In the *Pickwick Papers*, Dickens rejects the very notion of a child being able to inherit acquired characteristics, so that Joe could not be the son nor the father of obese men. Joe inhabits his own world and is neither degenerate nor the son of degenerates.

In 1893 *The Lancet* (citing an American case study) reports on a "case of narcolepsy."[22] A soldier who has regularly fallen asleep is accused of dereliction of duty because he has fallen asleep at his post. It is revealed that he seemed "well nourished and all his organs were apparently healthy. Mentally he did not seem to be lacking, although 'not very bright' best described his condition." He had fallen asleep on horseback while on parade as well as frequently falling "asleep at meals, on one occasion with a spoon in his mouth." His treatment was to put him on light duty. "Later he was placed on duty in the kitchen [where] he fell asleep and let the fire out and so delayed the meal." The author of the note concluded: "We have sometimes wondered whether Dickens had any knowledge of this as a distinct pathological condition when he described his immortal Fat Boy in 'Pickwick'." Dickens' character seems the appropriate reference for the readers of *The Lancet* to understand the nature of the soldier's ailment and narcolepsy seems the appropriate diagnosis for the Fat Boy's dilemma. Here too the mental acuity of the soldier seems to play a role in his diagnosis. He is not very bright and that seems to be part of the diagnostic category of narcolepsy. Being diagnosed with a disease, he is found innocent of a very serious breach of military discipline and transformed into a case that needs treatment.

Dickens' Fat Boy seems to form the basis for comparison in all cases. When in 1904 the parents of "The Fat Boy of Peckham," Johnnie Trundley, a 5½-year-old weighing 8 stones 5 lb., are accused of violating the "Act for the Prevention of Cruelty to Children" (1894) by exhibiting him as a freak, it is Dickens' character to whom the comparison is made.[23] The author of an editorial in *The Lancet* account notes, "Every traveling showman

would testify that obesity has always been as highly appreci-
ated by the public as abnormal stature, and the youthful
Trundley has had the advantage, or disadvantage, of living in
an age in which notoriety is easily achieved." But his celebrity,
the author notes, pales in comparison to the "heroes of fiction
[who] have the advantage in the matter of lasting glory and the
names of Daniel Lambert and the Fat Boy of Peckham sink into
insignificance beside those of Falstaff and the Fat Boy in 'Pickwick.'" Visibility as the ultimate case study of childhood
obesity is assured through the medium of literature.

In an account written by William Ord at the close of the
nineteenth century, the visibility still attendant to Dickens'
character appears in a case of obesity associated with hypothyroidism.[24] Ord provides an easy reference as to how one of his
patients is imagined as Dickens' Fat Boy Joe. His patient, a
30-year-old waiter, is admitted to St. Thomas' Hospital in
London in 1892 suffering from the end stages of the disease.
Diagnosed some six years earlier he had developed a set of both
psychological and physiological symptoms: "He began at first
to feel heavy, dull, and depressed, and became clumsy especially with his hands ... His abdomen and body generally began
to swell and his face became round, puffy, and yellowish-
brown with flushed cheeks, earning for him the nickname of
'The Fat Boy in *Pickwick*,' which replaced the nickname of 'Skin
and Buttons' which had before the illness been bestowed upon
him on account of his pale and hollow-eyed countenance." He
developed a "sort of Mongolian change of physiognomy."[25]
That there were specific physiognomic manifestations associated with hypothyroidism, the underproduction of thyroid
hormone, was well-known. Treated with thyroid extract, the
patients' symptoms diminished and he was able to return to

work even though he seemed clumsier at his job as a waiter than previously. The case had a negative outcome as the patient stopped coming to the clinic for the thyroid extract and eventually became an alcoholic, dying of symptoms associated with his disease in 1895. Ord's case study notes that the patient's nickname seemed to fit both his mental and physiological state. Joe was becoming a case of obesity defined as a disease of the body but hypothyroidism, with its diminished mental capacity, seemed not sufficient a cause to explain the power of the character.

With the shift in the explanation of childhood obesity to a focus on the endocrine system, Dickens' Fat Boy becomes a case of Froehlich's syndrome (an endocrine abnormality, caused by such things as a pituitary tumor or damage to the hypothalamus that reduce the production of specific hormones) rather than of thyroid insufficiency. The reason for this lies in the initial, yet deceptive, image of the asexuality of the Fat Boy, a quality not ascribed to the traditional definition of hypothyroidism (or indeed of goiter in its historical construction). By 1953, E. Watson-Williams dismisses "the well-known but irrelevant case of endocrine obesity recorded by Dickens."[26] However, the endocrine error is not hypothyroidism but an error of the pituitary gland. The Fat Boy becomes the test case in this battle of the various bodily causes of obesity. As early as 1922, H. Letheby Tidy had diagnosed Joe as a case of hypopituitarism (or Froehlich's syndrome) or, as he called it, stressing its sexual dimension, "dystrophia adiposogenitalis."[27] In addition to its onset before puberty in the form of morbid obesity ("adiposity"), other salient results of the low production of the pituitary hormone are deficiency of growth and "genital dystrophy or atrophy." The Fat Boy can have no desire because his sexual development is stunted! But, Watson-Williams observes, this does not impact on his awareness of the world or his innate intelligence. His face seems to deny this awareness. This type of hypopituitarism "may produce the appearance which was described...as the 'pudding-face type.'"[28] And yet this type, exemplified by Joe, is neither intellectually nor *emotionally* retarded. "Many of the famous Fat Boys have belonged to this group; the Fat Boy in Pickwick may be considered to be an example, and Dickens was by no means inaccurate in picturing him as possessing an acute intelligence in his waking moments." Joe is suffering from a childhood somatic illness, not from a weakness of the will or mind. His sexual desire is also "normal" even though his body may not be. He has now become a biological case study with a more limited and specific cause, unlike the "Hindoo Fat Boy" reported some seventy-five years earlier.

It is in the world of mid-twentieth-century pulmonary medicine that the conflict between the psychological and the metabolic causes of obesity, at least in regards to the "Fat Boy," seems to be resolved. This is the creation of the "Pickwick Syndrome,"[29] a term coined by C. Sidney Burwell and his colleagues at Harvard in 1956.[30] This is a form of obstructive sleep apnea syndrome, the condition by which people stop breathing for very short intervals of time during their normal sleep periods. Patients have a marked loss of oxygen in the blood system and ongoing lethargy while awake because of their inability to get any restful sleep. Burwell's paper presented a single case study of the "association of obesity, somnolence, polycythemia, and excessive appetite" and defined a new syndrome. Despite its name, the eponymous figure is, not to any one's surprise, Charles Dickens' Mr. Samuel Pickwick from *The Pickwick Papers* (1836–7), but rather Mr. Wardle's "Fat Boy," Joe.

Instead of considering the societal and stigmatizing ramifications of obesity, as did Dickens, Burwell sees Joe solely in terms of his pathophysiology and not in terms of the morality read into his body. Burwell strengthens his argument that Joe is a case study by citing William Wadd's early-nineteenth-century medical account of "corpulence." There have been claims of a greater antiquity for this syndrome.[31] It is the case of "a country tradesman aged about 30, of a short stature and naturally of a fresh, sanguine complexion and very fat…" who was suffering from the combination of symptoms that Burwell finds in Joe. The Burwell article presents a *single* case study of a man, 51 years old, 5 feet 5 inches tall, who weighed 263 pounds. The salient incident in this patient's life that brought him to the hospital was the fact that he fell asleep during a poker game while holding three aces and two kings! His was neither an error of intelligence (he recognized after the fact what he had done) nor an inappropriate emotional response. He is a somatic Fat Boy. In a completely phenomenological description of the case, Burwell and his colleagues see excessive eating as both the cause and a symptom, but avoid any discussion of the cause of his patient's (and Joe's) illness. Burwell's case is that of an adult.[32] The medical community adopted the term "Pickwickian syndrome" after 1960 when two remarkably similar cases to that in the literature were reported in children.[33]

Contemporary psychoanalysis was at the height of its American prominence in the 1950s. The debate about the nature of Joe's illness was engaged by the psychiatrist, psychoanalyst, and popular writer on body image Hilde Bruch, (1904–84). She attempted to counter such rather mechanistic readings of the

Fat Boy. In her classic study, *Eating Disorders* (1973), Bruch too cites Dickens, employing the passage where Joe awakens abruptly when he is offered food:

> (Sundry taps on the head with a stick, and the fat boy, with some difficulty, roused from his lethargy.) "Come, hand in the eatables."
> There was something in the sound of the last word which roused the unctuous boy. He jumped up, and the leaden eyes which twinkled behind his mountainous cheeks leered horribly upon the food as he unpacked it from the basket.
> "Now make haste," said Mr. Wardle; for the fat boy was hanging fondly over a capon, which he seemed wholly unable to part with. The boy sighed deeply, and, bestowing an ardent gaze upon its plumpness, unwillingly consigned it to his master.[34]

She continues, "During the 1930s and the 1940s, Joe's behavior was often cited as evidence of the sleepiness of the pituitary type of obesity. During the 1950s the eponym "Pickwickian Syndrome" was given to the clinical picture of extreme obesity associated with alveolar hypoventilation and hypoxic somnolence. Yet I doubt Joe suffered from it. I have never seen an organically determined somnolence in which one word had such a vitalizing influence."[35] Bruch dismisses all of the earlier work that defined Joe's mental and physical state as the result of a purely metabolic error. This was the general state of the medical understanding of obesity in the 1940s when she began her work.

Her interest in obesity actually builds on her own dissertation written in 1928, where character and body size are clearly linked. Her image of a lazy, stupid fat child comes to be more differentiated in her later reading of Joe. Her image, as with her earlier work in Weimar Germany, provides Joe (and all fat children, real or imagined) with a family that cannot love them as the cause of their obesity.

In the twenty-first century, the pendulum has swung very much in the other direction. Obesity has again become defined as physiological rather than psychological. In the 1990s this focus has been the function of the obesity hormone, leptin, in weight regulation in mice genetically created in the laboratory as "obese mice."[36] In 2006 the French researcher Claudio Rabec presented a paper on the "New Adventures of Mr. Pickwick" in which he reanimates "Fat Joe." There he documents that, "Leptin seems to have miscellaneous effects on respiratory function in obesity."[37] With this he provides a "pathophysiological explanation to the 'phenotype' of Joe, 'this fat red-faced boy, who snores as he waits at table, falls asleep easily and then stops breathing'." All of the respiratory problems that defined obesity at mid-century were simply the result of the underproduction of a specific hormone. Joe is a massive sufferer from the underproduction of leptin. To cure him, just provide him with a shot of leptin. (As an aside, this does not seem actually to work in practice with obese individuals except for the tiniest fraction of those who suffer from very specific and very limited genetic error. Clearly, if it were the cause of obesity and the attendant somatic ills, the obesity epidemic could be cured with an injection.) But of course the opposite is also true today: an Italian research team has recently used "Fat Joe" as the model for the retrospective diagnosis of "obstructive sleep apnea syndrome" in the widest range of historical figures, including Napoleon Bonaparte, Queen Victoria, and Franklin D. Roosevelt (only Victoria became obese in her old age).[38] By 2007 Dickens' character is again revived as a somatic case: "a fat young boy called Joe who eats and sleeps excessively and has trouble waking up. Joe is a 'red-faced boy' (perhaps suffering from polycythemia) with 'mountainous cheeks' and dropsy (perhaps a clinical sign of heart failure), who snores loudly and has a bizarre personality."[39] "Fat Joe" is now a case study in the new medical culture of obesity, where physical states are the *cause* of psychological disorders. This is the antithesis of the psychological reading of Joe's obesity.

Of course, retrospective diagnosis using fictional characters as one's case study provides a very high degree of certainty, since fiction (as we have seen) lends itself to infinite reinterpretations. Joe remains the classic obese patient and his "disease" is shaped to fit the latest theories about the meaning and function of obesity. But Joe himself was the reinvention of an older trope that connected body size with being "drowsy in the day; the repletion still increases, and their nights begin to grow restless; their sleep afterwards becomes disturbed with frightful dreams of battles."[40] Thus states Hippocrates (or at least the Hippocratic corpus) on overweight men in the fourth century BCE. But Joe's Victorian dreams linger on food and sex, not battle, very different fantasies attributed to the psyche of the obese. As we shall see, the question of what obesity means in medicine remains as fraught today in our age of "globesity" as it has in the past.

II

OBESITY FROM THE ANCIENTS TO THE BEGINNING OF THE MODERN AGE

Obesity has a role in all of the ancient medical systems in the West. In the ancient world, obesity is a case study that illustrates how illness was intrinsically understood as part of a relationship of the human being to the totality of the universe, including the divine. Such a holistic view was slowly replaced in the Enlightenment with the understanding of disease that sees obesity as a problem of the body and therefore responsive to the knowledge of the medical practitioner. For the ancient world, the control of the body and its weight was an intrinsic part of religious belief. The ancient Greeks saw food as part of a complex web that connected human beings and the gods through the humors.

In ancient Greek medicine, as the Hippocratic author of *On Ancient Medicine* famously claimed, it is physicians and not philosophers who understand best the nature of man. In ancient Greece, fat as a pathological category appears in texts ascribed to Hippocrates (c. 440–370 BCE). Hippocrates, or at least as attributed to him in the approximately sixty texts of the Hippocratic corpus, based his notion of health and illness on the balance of the humors, the *chymoi*. According to this

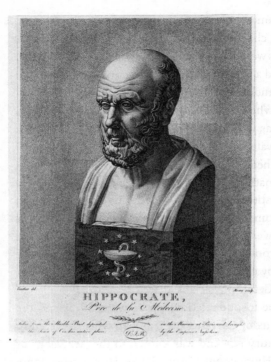

HIPPOCRATE,
Père de la Médecine

4. Hippocrates. Engraving after a marble bust of Hippocrates; by A. M. Cou, n.d. (*Wellcome Collection*)

view, these four crucial bodily fluids, blood, yellow bile, black bile, and phlegm, were found in all individuals, and produced health when in balance and illness when one dominated over the others. They also produced the visible aspects of the body that could be measured by the physician: blood made the body hot and wet; choler, hot and dry; black bile, cold and dry; and phlegm, cold and wet. They were also correlated to the four ages of man—infancy, youth, adulthood, and old age—and to the essential aspects of the world—air, fire, earth, and water. The physician could intervene to alter the domination of one or the other humors, often with lifestyle or regimen changes, which entailed changing the food or activities of the patient. But the humors were also the key to bodily shape and physique. Thus, if one had a natural predisposition to phlegm it resulted in fat. Each humor also determined temperament; the phlegmatic person (who was also fat) was pale, lazy, inert, and cool in character—as well as, of course, phlegmatic. Phlegm was "naturally" of water and of old age.

In humoral theory, fat could either be a sign of indisposition with the domination of phlegm to be treated by hot and dry foods or a constitutional status (as in aging), in which one's phlegmatic nature could be mitigated but not altered. In the first case, one was a fat patient, but not in the second. Greek medicine was rooted in the practice of *diatetica*, the diet as the primary therapy or, to use a more modern phrase, "eating as healing." The Greek physicians therefore also believed that there was a one-to-one relationship between foods and the effects. Dionysus of Carystus (in Euboea), who practiced in the fourth century BCE and was known to the Athenians as the "younger Hippocrates," argued like Hippocrates for a completely causal relationship in dietetics. Certain foods were not only healthful but also curative, just as a surfeit of others were the cause of illness, and central among those illnesses was obesity.

For the followers of Hippocrates, fat and thin could be either "natural" antitheses or signs of illness in terms of the balance and unbalance of the humors. Thus, fat reflects the pathological state of the body caused by imbalance. For the patient who is fat as a sign of disease, there is also a clear distinction between fat men and fat women: "When unnaturally fat women cannot conceive, it is because the fat presses the mouth of the womb, and conception is impossible until they grow thinner."[1] But men "who are constitutionally very fat are more apt to die quickly than those who are thin,"[2] abandoning their families and their role in society, both paramount responsibilities in the ancient world. In all cases, extreme fat falls in the realm of medicine: "Repletion too, carried to extremes, is perilous," he observes.[3] Hippocrates does acknowledge that corpulence gave one a slight advantage against febrile diseases, but it was greatly outweighed by the pathological effects. The cure was eating after "exercise and while still panting from fatigue and with no other refreshment before meals except wine, diluted and slightly cold. They should, moreover, eat only once a day and take no baths and sleep on a hard bed and walk naked as long as possible." Quite literally a Spartan regime, as this was the way that the Spartan society deemed its citizens to act!

Greek medicine, in seeing the dominance of phlegm as pathology, also evolved the concept of *polysarkia*, too much flesh. This is a term reintroduced into Roman medicine by the North African Caelius Aurelianus in the fifth century CE in his *De morbis acutis et chronicis*. Polysarkia was the result of the imbalance of the humors, but also a quality of temperament. Thus the lazy, phlegmatic person also consumes too much food. They live in a concomitant state of slothfulness and stupidity. Such people violated the principle of constraint in all things. Constraint, Socrates frequently reminded his listeners, is the greatest good and in complex ways the obese male violates this dictum.

The line that the Hippocratic corpus assumes between acceptable fat and excessive fat (extreme repletion) is the difference between life and death. In Aristotle's essay on longevity, fat is the quality that preserves warmth. Animals (including human beings) are "naturally moist and warm, and life too is of this nature, whereas old age is cold and dry, and so is a dead body."(*Aristotle*, "On Length and Shortness of Life").⁴ Aristotle (384–322 BCE) continues: "Fatty things are not liable to decay because they contain air...air like fire does not become corrupt."⁵ "Bloodless" animals are protected by their fat: "In animals the fat is sweet; for this reason, bees are longer lived than other larger animals."⁶ Here too the line is assumed between acceptable "fatness" and pathological obesity.

Strength, health, and beauty are the "virtues" of the classical Greek body. It is no accident that one of the most important commentators on diet of the ancient world was Herodicus of Selymbria, a trainer of athletes, who used gymnastics to cure his own fat body. Hippocrates had stressed that, "In athletes a perfect condition that is at its highest pitch is treacherous. Such conditions cannot remain the same or be at rest, and, change for the better being impossible, the only possible change is for the worse. For this reason it is an advantage to reduce the fine embonpoint quickly, in order that the body may make a fresh beginning of growth."⁷ Here it is the professional *athletae* who competed in the games, rather than the *agonistae*—those who sought health and strength through gymnastics—who need to be thin. And that cure for the fat body was diet and exercise.

Early Roman medicine, following the lead of classical Greek medicine, saw obesity as a sign of illness. This was best articulated in the works of Aulus Cornelius Celsus (c. 25 BCE–c. 50 CE) the Roman encyclopedist, known for his extant medical work, *De Medicina*, the only surviving section of a much larger encyclopedia of general knowledge. Celsus and Roman medicine used the term *obesitas*, a term also used by the Latin poet Suetonius. Celsus argued, however, that the body tended

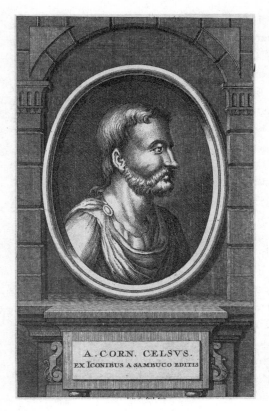

A . CORN. CELSVS.
EX ICONIBUS A SAMBUCO EDITIS

5. A. Cornelius
Celsus. Engraving
by J. van der Spyk,
n.d. (*Wellcome
Collection*)

toward fat naturally. Nevertheless, too much weight was a sign
of disease. "The obese, many of them, are throttled by acute
diseases and difficult breathing; they die often suddenly, which
rarely happens in the thinner person."[8] In treating extra weight,
he suggests tepid saltwater baths, hard exercise, food of an
austere kind, and restricted sleep. Yet he recognized the need
to indulge in excess as part of the social fabric of the table.
Moderation indeed but never to excess!

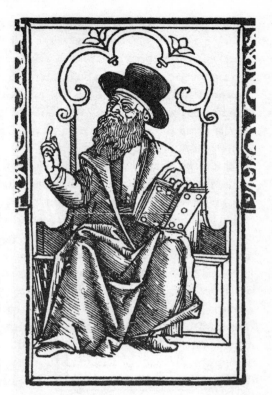

6. Galen, from
*Therapeutica lib.
XIV. Therapeutica
ad Glauconem* lib.
II. (Venice: Z.
Callierges for N.
Blastus, 1500).
(*Wellcome
Collection*)

More important is the shift in Roman medicine, which takes place in the first century when Galen (129–c. 216 CE) began to rethink the basic categories of Hippocratic medicine. He dismissed mere "empiricism" as per the Hippocratic method and demanded that there be a theoretical underpinning to medical knowledge. While the Hippocratic physicians used foodstuffs to treat the imbalance of the humors, Galen saw the natural world as the very source of the illness from which human beings suffer. The core concept remains the humors; Galen's dictum is that, "It is always the case that everything superfluous in the body runs to the weakest site and produces effect in them according to its own nature."⁹ For Galen, what is common in all the diseases is "*plethos*," an excess of bad blood, blood mixed with "residues," which, if not excreted, would wander about the body, settle in weak parts, and there cause "putrefaction."

Yet it is the external world that provides the source of such residues. It is not the weak will of the phlegmatic individual that leads to *polysarkia* (too much flesh), but the very nature of the food itself. For Galen in his *On the Fat and Lean Mode of Life*, the causes of illness lie in those things that are "non-natural," (i.e., not the humors) *res contra naturum*: *aer* (light and air), *cibus et portus* (food and drink), *motus et quies* (movement and rest), *somnux et vigilia* (sleeping and waking), *exkreta et sekreta* (metabolism), and *affectus animi* (affect). This was an argument that made "nurture" equivalent to "nature." But he always stressed that obesity and its reduction was in the hands of the patient, who should always be in control of their indulgences. In his *De Alimentorum Facultatibus* (*On the Nature of Foods*), Galen suggests "quick exercise" as a cure for obesity. He provides food, "but not of a very nourishing description," to be consumed only after exercise. He argued that a "sufficiently stout patient [could become] moderately thin in a short time by running and massages."¹⁰ The cause of obesity lies in the natural products of the world consumed in excess. His work was as much for the educated lay reader as for the medical professional. Galen provides clear guidance about what is good to eat and what is not. His first book deals with "starchy" products of nature and what foods result from them, the second with fruits and vegetables, and the third with animal products.

Galen's approach is culinary as well as medical; he suggests how food should be best and most tastefully prepared. His focus is both on treating the ill and preserving the healthy. All foods, according to Galen, are necessary and natural but used improperly they can create illness.

Following Galen, the Alexandrian physician Paul of Aegina (625?–690?) in the seventh century saw obesity as a problem only when it is "immoderate." Since "warm temperament renders the body lean," it is this state that should be created in fat people. "Active exercise, an attenuated regimen, medicines of the same class, and mental anxiety bring on the dry temperament, and thereby render the body lean."[11] He also recommends that diuretics and small amounts of food (in proportion to exercise taken and preferably only once a day) should be undertaken.

The Romans incorporated diet as a classical therapy along with exercise to treat obesity. The key to all of the diets suggested was the Greek concept of a moderate reduction of foodstuffs complemented by exercise and some herbal treatments. In general, Galenic medicine saw "food as therapy," but it also was concerned with questions of food as preserving health and life.

On the other side of the Mediterranean, the Jews were also concerned with the meanings associated with food, if not with obesity. The Bible (Old Testament, Tanach) contains a long series of prohibitions concerning food, which also connect food consumption with the divine. Prohibited are certain foods from any animal that does not have both cloven hooves and chew its cud (pigs)[12] or fish or seafood that does not have fins and scales (sturgeon or shrimp),[13] as well as rules concerning the combinations of foods that may be eaten.

Added to these rules are specific laws concerning slaughter and the preparation of meat.[14] Given the focus of the Jews on diet, it is surprising how little emphasis Jews placed on the representation of the overweight body. Such a body is evoked by the biblical figure of Eglon, King of Moab, who oppressed the children of Israel for eighteen years. His fat (*ish bari me'od*) body was destroyed by the left-handed hero Ehud.[15] Indeed, it is even described how Eglon's fat closed about the blade when he was pierced. Ehud smuggles his sword into the presence of the king by wearing it on the "wrong side," at least the wrong side for right-handers. He is categorized as treacherous and sneaky. As for the fat king, his guards do not even notice that he has been disemboweled until they smell his feces. In the commentaries on the Holy Writ, the Talmud, the fat body was a deviant one, but not particularly a dangerous one. Rather, there is a sort of fascination with it. The Talmud even asks whether very fat men, such as Rabbis Ishmael ben Yose and Eleazar ben Simeon (end of the second century) could ever reproduce because of their huge bellies. But Jewish attitudes toward such obesity were clearly defined by the model of the lack of self-control. Not yet a "sin," it was a sign of the lack of self-discipline appropriate for a real man, a real scholar, and could be punished.

For Jewish physicians in the post-Temple age, the notion of obesity and cure becomes a concern. The Jewish physician Isaac Judaeus a.k.a. Abu Ya'kub ibn Sulaiman Alisr'ili (before 832–932 CE), was born in Egypt and had his major impact in Tunis where he died. As a student of 'Ishak ibn 'Amran al-Baghdadi, he incorporated the traditions of Greek medicine as understood by contemporary Jewish and Muslim physicians. He was court physician to the last Aghiabite prince,

Ziyadat Allah, and in 909 CE became the official physician to the Fatimid Caliph Ubaid Allah al-Mahdi and, as such, had enormous influence in the medical world of his day. He was the author of, among many other medical works, a treatise on disease and its cures, *Kitab al-adwiya al-mufrada wal-aghdhiya*, the last three sections of which were translated into Latin as *De diaetis particularibus*. This was the first dedicated book on dieting published in Europe. His works' initial impact on Christian Europe came with their translation into Latin in 1087 by Constantine of Carthage (a.k.a. the African), who claimed that he had written the works himself. His dieting book was then translated into Hebrew from the Latin as *Sefer ha-Ma'akalim* and was first published from a manuscript in Padua in 1484. This book was immediately translated into the vernacular, and a German translation by Valentin Schwendes appeared in 1498. It was only in 1515 that these works were finally attributed to Isaac Judaeus, who was one of the most influential interpreters of Greek medical knowledge for the Muslim world. Many of his works were written in Arabic as well as Hebrew.

In the classic work on dietetics of the twelfth century, Iberian physician-philosopher Maimonides' the *Regimen of Health*, there is no sense that obesity was a moral or even a medical problem (at least for the rulers for whom he wrote), while he notes sexual overexertion as one. However, it was still viewed as an important health issue with repercussions on the body of the individual; he treated the condition of "obese old men" with medication, exercise, massage, and baths. His work provides a synthesis of Galenic medicine and the work of the Arabic physician Ibn Sina (Avicenna, 980–1037), whose *Kitah al-Quanun* or *The Canon* includes a detailed discussion of obesity in its fourth book. His treatment was an appetite suppressant made of almonds and beef suet, marsh-mallow root, and oil of violets, taken for ten days to abate hunger.

Such views developed during the Jewish Diaspora in Muslim and Christian Europe. The notion that our bodies are God's temples was also part and parcel of Western Christianity, beginning with Paul (who demanded that we control our venal appetites). (It thus also became part of both rabbinic Judaism and Islam.) Such a view saw the obese and unhealthy body as a sign of man's faulty relationship with God and with God's complex world and named gluttony as one of the seven deadly sins.

Health becomes one of the powerful metaphors in early Christianity, especially in terms of the relationship between the newly healthy body of the Christian and the sick body of the Jew. Jesus' cures are his most powerful miracles. With the establishment of early Christianity (most readily seen in St. Augustine's *Confessions*) the submission to the temptation to overeat was written on the body in the form of fat. "*Gula*" (gluttony) is one of the seven deadly sins of the early Church. In many ways, it is the most difficult of the deadly sins to combat.

Augustine (354–430), the Bishop of Hippo in North Africa, struggled against lust and begged for chastity in his early youth: "But I, wretched, most wretched, in the very commencement of my early youth, had begged chastity of Thee, and said, 'Give me chastity and continency, only not yet.'" When he turned 16, Augustine moved to Carthage where again he was plagued by desire: "Where there seethed all around me a cauldron of lawless loves. I loved not yet, yet I loved to love, and out of a deep-seated want, I hated myself for wanting not. I sought what I might love, in love with loving, and I hated safety … To love then, and to be beloved, was sweet to me; but more, when

I obtained to enjoy the person I loved. I defiled, therefore, the spring of friendship with the filth of concupiscence, and I beclouded its brightness with the hell of lustfulness." Yet he writes that he struggles each day with the desire to eat and to drink even more that he does with sexual lust: "In the midst of these temptations I struggle daily against greed for food and drink. This is not an evil which I can decide once and for all to repudiate and never to embrace again, as I was able to do with fornication."[16] For the seduction of food and what it signifies, the fat body haunts Augustine's sense of himself. He sees food as both necessary for health and a force for healing, but only in strict limits: "I look upon food as a medicine. But the snare of concupiscence awaits me in the very process of passing from the discomfort of hunger to the contentment, which comes when satisfied. For the process itself is a pleasure and there is no other means of satisfying hunger except the one, which we are obliged to take...Health and enjoyment have not the same requirement." The desire for food is itself the Devil present in the body. He cites Paul in that "we gain nothing by eating, lose nothing by abstaining."[17] This is a basic struggle to control desire and the very form of the body. Augustine makes the ideal body the body divine, much as in the Platonic notion of beauty it is beyond the material.

In his *City of God*, Augustine links the carnal pleasures of the flesh with sins of the soul. They are the same. He condemns with equal verve the Epicurean philosophers who "live after the flesh, because they place man's highest good in bodily pleasure" and the Stoics, "who place the supreme good of men in the soul, live after the spirit." The Epicureans also claim that, "Pleasure is very largely a matter of physical health," and the Stoics that "only the wise are beautiful."[18] Augustine quotes

Paul over and over again on the need to control carnality and the fallen nature of the soul. There is a compelling case for understanding the Pauline letters themselves as allegorical. Paul's allegory presents linked pairs such as, flesh–spirit, literal–figurative, signifier–signified, in which the first element points to the privileged, second element. And so, for Paul, the Torah points only to the fulfillment of its prophecy of the coming Messiah in Christ. The ideal body can be found only in heaven when he describes heavenly bodies as possessing "a wondrous ease of movement, a wondrous lightness." Here the image of the perfectly light and slim body of the divine body is in contrast to the mortal and sinful one.

The crucial early Christian text is again from Paul's letters: "knowledge puffs up, but love builds up."[19] Fat, as a sign of gluttony, is a reflection of prideful nature of humans. It is often linked to *acedia*, sloth, the deadly sin that is also part of the tradition of the representation of madness in the West. The puffed-up body is also the spirit that is so unwilling to act as to be a sign of moral decay and mental instability. For Augustine it is his body, in which all desires seem confused and interchangeable. It is the body most at risk from inaction and desire.

Here it is St. Thomas Aquinas (1225–74) who must rethink these limitations in Pauline terms when he preaches that, "Meditating upon all these things, let us not give our minds to delights, but to what is the end of delights. Here on earth it is excrement and obesity, hereafter it is fire and the worm."[20] If for Paul all human beings are damned by their flesh, Aquinas needs to stress this once again, by seeing us trapped in our fallen bodies by our natural functions—eating and excreting. Indeed, he provides a list of gluttony in its widest forms:

Praepropere	Eating too soon,
Laute	Eating too expensively,
Nimis	Eating too much,
Ardenter	Eating too eagerly,
Studiose	Eating too daintily,
Forente	Eating wildly.

And yet it is Saint Teresa who says, that the soul "finds everything cooked and eaten for it; it has only to enjoy its nourishment."[21] This is now the pure food of the spirit, not of the flesh.

In the medical school at Salerno in the thirteenth century, the standard textbook of medicine, the *Regimen sanitatis salernitanum*—the *Salernitan Regime of Health*—was composed. A book of verses attributed to Arnald of Villanova (1240–1311), it provided practical guidelines for good living, but also definitions of the healthy and pathological bodies. Extraordinarily popular, it summarized and informed much of the later views of obesity. In a seventeenth-century English translation, it provided a snapshot of the humoral obese body in the light of the medieval reception of Greek medicine:

> Men that be flegmatik, are weak of nature,
> Most commonly of thick and stubbed stature.
> And fatnesse overtaketh them amain,
> For they are slothfull, and can take no pain.
> Their fences are but dull, shallow and slow,
> Much given to sleep, whence can no goodnesse grow,
> They often spet: yet natures kind direction,
> Hath blest them with a competent complexion.[22]

Thus, phlegmatic fat persons cannot stand pain; they suffer from character flaws and are lazy, and non-productive. But there is also a healthy fat that dines on:

> Sweet wine, delicious meats, eggs that are rare
> Over ripe figs and raisins, these appear.
> To make the body fat, and nourish nature,
> Procuring corpulence, and growth of stature.[23]

Corpulence is not obesity. This fat can itself become diseased but is of a different nature than the inherent obesity of the phlegmatic body because it came from a different source. Food can cause illness, as Galen states, but there is also a "healthy" fat that is the result of eating without overindulgence. The cure for overindulgence is to eat foods with the antithetical humoral traits as the fat person. Thus, drinking vinegar (which is dry and cool) as therapy for the obese body (wet and cool), "unto fat folks, greatly doth no good."[24] You need to eat the opposite to that which has made you fat.

The sixteenth-century Italian physician, Gerolamo Mercuriale, also stresses that obesity is the result of internal and external factors, paraphrasing Galen. Yet he also understands that the obese are not all stupid; indeed, they can be as intellectual as the thin person. Any given person can be born with the tendency toward *obesitas*. But *adventitia*, the acquired fat of a dissolute life, makes the mind crude. It is the result of an oily blood that turns to fat. His contemporary, Tommaso Minadoi, follows Galen's theory of the temperaments, seeing damp and cold as the origin of fat. Such people are born, not made; they are soft, hairless, pale, and cold. Those who become fat are quite different. They are of a reddish complexion, hairy, have hard rather than soft flesh. They suffer from a constant hunger that drives them to become fat. Such theories build on the notion of a "natural" and an "unnatural" obesity, which demand different types of diet.

The moral lessons associated with obesity in the world of ancient medicine are an inherent part of the medical understanding of this state through the beginning of the modern world. Science is part of religion, as it is seen as a means of understanding the complexity of human health and illness within a world view that does not separate the human from the divine. By the sixteenth century, we begin to see that the moral meanings associated with the overly large body are now understood in ways that stress the political and social meanings of health and illness and are seemingly becoming separated from notions of the divine. The scientific revolution of the Renaissance, such as Galileo's understanding of the physics of the solar system, begins to shape the medical and popular understanding of obesity.

III

OBESITY FROM THE RENAISSANCE TO THE ENLIGHTENMENT

By the Renaissance, the Christian understanding of gluttony as the wellspring of obesity comes into conflict with a new scientific understanding of obesity. The Venetian, Alvise Luigi Cornaro (c. 1467–1566), is certainly the earliest and most influential author of the literature dealing with obesity and its cure written during the Italian Renaissance. Cornaro is read in every epoch following the Renaissance and still has a readership today. His elegantly written Italian text, *Discorsi della vita sobria*, variously in English translated as the *Discourses on a Sober Life*, the *Art of Living Long* and also the *Temperate Life*, first appeared in 1558. Begun in 1550 when he was 83, the final instalment appeared when he was 95. It became an instant best-seller and remains in print today.

Cornaro confesses to the reader that at middle age, he was dissipated by forty years of gluttony and overindulgence in sensual pleasures. He was at death's door. For him gluttony was a killer, not merely a sin, for it "kills every year…as great a number as would perish during the time of a most dreadful pestilence, or by the sword or fire of many bloody wars!"[1] In the depths of his illness, he turned to the physicians. They advised

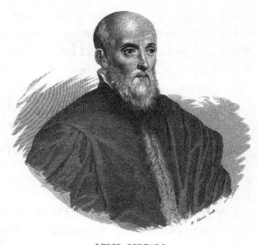

LUIGI CORNARO
Dal ritratto dipinto da Tiziano

7. Luigi Cornaro. Engraving by F. Clerici. (*Wellcome Collection*)

him to be temperate. He thus cured his obese body through a strict limitation of his diet. While the cure is for him proof of the beneficence of God, it is equally proof that living longer allows one to develop those "splendid gifts of intellect and noble qualities of heart,"[2] which can evolve once the demands and desires of youth are met. In a sense, the evidence for God's grace and the best use of his gifts comes at the end of life. It is a "natural death" that comes at the time when one's vital powers have diminished and one dies well—peacefully and without struggle.

Cornaro's text is a handbook for a good life (and death). Its power lies in its autobiographical, indeed, confessional mode, which echoes Augustine. He observes, and carefully chronicles, his symptoms as a younger man from his perspective as an old, healthy, thin man. He was certainly ill with many of the diseases attributed to obesity in the Galenic tradition: "I had pains in the stomach, frequent pains in the side, symptoms of gout, and, still worse, a low fever that was almost continuous; but I suffered especially from disorder of the stomach, and from an unquenchable thirst."[3] But he also lost his ability to reject temptation, having become addicted to eating and drinking. He turned to the physicians whose advice was quite clear; they "declared there was but one remedy left for my ills—a remedy which would surely conquer them, provided I would make up my mind to apply it and persevere in its use. That remedy was the temperate and orderly life."[4] This is what the physicians admonished and what the patient followed to success.

Sobriety after a life of indulgence is a cure for the physical effects of obesity, not obesity itself. Cornaro sees himself as typical of the men of his age. The riches of their lives have led to the brink of death as a result of what he identified as the three evil customs or sins widespread in sixteenth-century Italy: "adulation and ceremony…heresy and…intemperance."[5] Only through the good counsel of the doctors does he find a cure for all three. For gluttony is understood as the cause of the list of infirmities found in the fat man. The overindulgence of the man in his best years is the cause of his fat and his fat is the sign of his sick body. There is a strong moral tradition that owes its form to Paul and the Christian abnegation of the body. The society in which he lives, however, does not understand this simple rule:

> These false notions are due entirely to the force of habit, bred by men's senses and uncontrolled appetites. It is this craving to gratify the appetites which has allured and inebriated men to such a degree that, abandoning the path

of virtue, they have taken to following the one of vice—a road which leads them, though they see it not, to strange and fatal chronic infirmities through which they grow prematurely old. Before they reach the age of 40 their health has been completely worn out—just the reverse of what the temperate life once did for them. For this, before it was banished by the deadly habit of intemperance, invariably kept all its followers strong and healthy, even to the age of fourscore and upward.[6]

It is not knowledge of the world that cures, but simplicity and temperance. He bemoans the fact that, "Friends and associates, men endowed with splendid gifts of intellect and noble qualities of heart, who fall, in the prime of life, victims of this dread tyrant; men who, were they yet living, would be ornaments to the world, while their friendship and company would add to my enjoyment in the same proportion as I was caused sorrow by their loss."[7] He is now cured of his illnesses and fat by his strict regime. The world of simplicity may have its roots in the advice of physicians, but when Cornaro, at the age of 70, was in a carriage accident and dislocated an arm and leg, he rejected his physician's suggestion that he be bled. He was convinced that his now healthy body would heal itself and, according to his account, it did. As a result of his own diet, he believes he knows his body so well, that he is aware of what it needs to evince a cure.

Moderation is now his model for men to regain their manhood, a manhood defined by longevity. And Cornaro was long-lived. This indeed was the key to his claim on authenticity in writing his autobiographical text. After the beginning of the sixteenth century, this anxiety about premature death was heightened. Cornaro's rejection of excess in food parallels Augustine's anxiety that gluttony was even worse than sexual license, for one did not have to fornicate (to use Augustine's

41

concept) but one did have to eat. But what is excessive in the intake of nourishment for one man may not be for another. One can eat anything one wants but in moderation.

> I began to observe very diligently what kinds of food agreed with me. I determined, in the first place, to experiment with those, which were most agreeable to my palate, in order that I might learn if they were suited to my stomach and constitution. The proverb, "Whatever tastes good will nourish and strengthen," is generally regarded as embodying a truth, and is invoked, as a first principle, by those who are sensually inclined. In it I had hitherto firmly believed; but now I was resolved to test the matter, and find to what extent, if any, it was true. My experience, however, proved this saying to be false.[8]

Since we must eat, as Augustine noted, we cannot suffer only to eat those things that give us pleasure, for that will only make us more gluttonous. Appetite is but a form of desire. Cornaro translates this into the discourse of health and illness. Eat for pleasure and you will become ill. But it is also clear that the ability to eat exactly those things that he needs is linked with his idea that certain foods are simply healthy in and of themselves. (We know this type of argument from the claim that "Cows' milk is the perfect food," first made in the nineteenth century. Given the high rate of lactose intolerance in various populations across the world, it does not hold true, but try and persuade your mother of that.)

Those foods, such as meat and fish, clearly evoke the wealth that was part of the temptation of Cornaro's youth. A member of the powerful Cornaro family of Venice, he could earlier afford to be gluttonous and now he can afford to eat fish.

> Of meats, I eat veal, kid, and mutton. I eat fowls of all kind; as well as partridges and birds like the thrush. I also

partake of such saltwater fish as the goldney and the like; and, among the various freshwater kinds, the pike and others...Old persons, who, on account of poverty, cannot afford to indulge in all of these things, may maintain their lives with bread, bread soup, and eggs—foods that certainly cannot be wanting even to a poor man, unless he be one of the kind commonly known as good-for-nothing. Yet, even though the poor should eat nothing but bread, bread soup, and eggs, they must not take a greater quantity than can be easily digested; for they must, at all times, remember that he who is constantly faithful to the above-mentioned rules in regard to the quantity and quality of his food, cannot die except by simple dissolution and without illness.[9]

Cornaro resolved to restrict his diet drastically. Initially, it was reduced to a daily intake of twelve ounces of food and fourteen ounces of wine. Eventually, however, it was reduced to a single egg a day. However, he also understood the relationship between the outward manifestation of the body and its spirit. He resolved to control his temper and the "melancholy, hatred, and other passions of the soul, which all appear greatly to affect the body."[10] Assuming that he was in fact born in 1564 (contesting some accounts that claim his age at death was 103), Cornaro lived to be 98 and, according to his autobiography, it is the accomplishments in old age that reveal the character of man. He muses on what it is to be old and healthy. This is defined by his ability to work and to concentrate on questions of private as well as public health:

My greatest enjoyment, in the course of my journeys going and returning, is the contemplation of the beauty of the country and of the places through which I travel. Some of these are in the plains; others on the hills, near rivers or fountains; and all are made still more beautiful by the presence of many charming dwellings surrounded by delightful gardens. Nor are these my diversions and pleasures rendered less sweet and less precious through the failing of sight or my hearing, or because any one of my senses is not perfect; for they are all—thank God!—most perfect. This is true especially of my sense of taste; for I now find more true relish in the simple food I eat, wheresoever I may chance to be, than I formerly found in the most delicate dishes at the time of my intemperate life...With the greatest delight and satisfaction, also, do I behold the success of an undertaking highly important to our State; namely, the fitting for cultivation of its waste tracts of country, numerous as they were. This improvement was commenced at my suggestion; yet I had scarcely ventured to hope that I should live to see it, knowing, as I do, that republics are slow to begin enterprises of great importance. Nevertheless, I have lived to see it. And I myself was present with the members of the committee appointed to superintend the work, for two whole months, at the season of the greatest heat of summer, in those swampy places; nor was I ever disturbed either by fatigue or by any hardship I was obliged to incur. So great is the power of the orderly life which accompanies me wheresoever I may go! Furthermore, I cherish a firm hope that I shall live to witness not only the beginning but also the completion, of another enterprise, the success of which is no less important to our Venice: namely, the protection of our estuary...These are the true and important recreations, these comforts and pastimes, of my old age, which is much more to be prized than the old age or even the youth of other men; since it is free, by the grace of God, from all the perturbations of the soul and the infirmities of the body, and is not subject to any of those troubles which woefully torment so many young men and so many languid and utterly worn-out old men.[11]

Cornaro's autobiography is at its heart a handbook of dietetics to reform the fat body and turn him into a healthy and abstentious man who can in turn create a healthy world.

Medical theory regarding physical weight had begun to be developed by physicians such as the Venetian Sanctorius Sanctorius (1561–1636) in late sixteenth-century Padua. Sanctorius monitored his body weight for thirty years. He announced in his *De statica medicina* (1614) that what he consumed weighed more than what he excreted and assumed that the missing weight had been perspired, a sign of health. He, therefore, recommended the regular weighing of the body to promote health as a means of controlling excess weight. In his aphorisms, he also argued against too rapid weight gain or loss, for "When the body is one day of one weight, and another day of another, it argues an introduction of evil qualities." But he implied that too great a weight gain is itself pathological: "That weight, which is to any one such as that when he goes up some steep place, he feels himself lighter than he is wont, is the exact standard of good health."[12] Consistent weight and mobility define health, and the act of weighing oneself in public became a measure of public accountability for one's health.

By the seventeenth century, there was the first, modern creation of a specialized literature of "healthy" and "unhealthy" foods, such as Johann Sigismund Elsholtz' (1623–88) *Diaeteticon* (1682). His tabulation of every possible food and drink that was (or could be) consumed for its healthy and unhealthy properties had become a standard for the classification of foods. Indeed, he quotes Galen to the effect that every physician should become knowledgeable in the art of cooking. Toward the end of his book he advises on the appropriate diet for men—they should combine eating with work or exercise, such as fencing. He also ends his book with a warning, following Hippocrates, that the body of the athletic man can more easily age and become ill when he overeats.

The moral questions remained, but slowly were loosed from the overt religious rhetoric of obesity. The French essayist Jean de La Bruyère (1645–96) presents us a series of portraits of men who are types, or "characters," in 1688. Among them is Clito who "had, throughout his life, been concerned with two things alone: namely, dining at noon and supping at night; he seems born to digest; he has only one topic of conversation: he tells you what entrées were served at the last meal he was at, how many soups there were and what sort of soups."[13] He is "the arbiter of good things." But sadly, La Bruyère notes, "he was giving a dinner party on the day he died. Wherever he may be, he is eating, and if he should come back to this world, it would be to eat." The deadly sin of "gula" (gluttony) has become gourmandizing, but the result is the same—death.

By the eighteenth century, obesity comes to be a major concern of physicians. Giovanni Battista Morgagni, one of the founders of modern anatomical pathology, stated in 1761 quite clearly that fat was a major risk factor for disease and specifically fat within the omentum of the bowel.[14] But "fat" had meaning beyond the anatomical for the Enlightenment.

The German Physician Royal to the King of Prussia and the creator of the term "macrobiotic," Christoph Wilhelm Hufeland had captured in his extraordinarily popular *The Art of Prolonging Life* (1796) the "good" and "moral" aspects of the physical nature of man.[15] Fat is simply bad for Hufeland and the Enlighteners because most people eat much more than they need. "Immoderation" is one of the prime causes of early death.[16] Invoking the golden mean, eating too much and eating too richly will kill you. "The first thing which, in regard to diet, can act as a shortener of life, is *immoderation*."[17] Too much food, too "refined" food are the cause of the shortening of life. Food that tastes too good makes one eat too much. Simple is better than complex: "Eggs, milk, butter, and flour are each, used by itself, very easy of digestion; but when joined together, and formed into a fat, solid pudding, the produce will be extremely heavy and indigestible."[18] "People in a natural state…require few rules respecting their diet."[19]. Balance in diet is vital: vegetables and bread must be eaten with meat. Indeed, the avoidance of "flesh" and of wine is advocated.[20] Healthy is simple; simple is long life.

"Idleness" is also a cause.[21] Human beings have lost their natural ability to determine how much we need by childhood overindulgence. Natural man, notes Hufeland, in plowing the fields has purpose, exercise, and food appropriate to long life. "His son becomes a studious rake; and the proportion between countrymen and citizens seems daily to be diminished."[22] The fat child is now the father (and mother) of the fat adult. Indeed, Hufeland places at the very beginning of his list of things that will certainly cause early death—a "very warm, tender, and delicate education" in childhood in which children are stuffed "immoderately with food; and by coffee, chocolate, wine, spices, and such things…"[23] Not sin but middle class overindulgence begins to be seen as the force that creates fat boys. In the nineteenth century, the "science" of diet seems to replace the morals of diet. The hidden model remains the same: the normal, reasonable man is always contrasted with the Fat Boy and always to the Fat Boy's detriment. And the reward for the thin man is life, life extended (and if Augustine is to be believed, life eternal), while the fat person dies young and badly.

Immanuel Kant (1724–1804) reads Hufeland and answers him in print: his claim was that it is not the world but our perception of it that is at fault. And thus the battle lines of the modern diet wars are drawn: who will cure the obese sufferer? The physician or the psychologist? Kant, in his essay on "Overcoming Unpleasant Sensations by mere Reasoning" (1797), argued that dietetics could only become philosophy "when the mere power of reason in mankind, in overcoming sensations by a governing principle, determines their manner of living. On the other hand, when it endeavors to excite or avert these sensations, by external corporeal means, the art becomes merely empiric and mechanical."[24] This is his direct answer to Hufeland's empiricism. Hufeland had sent him his book on diet and longevity in the winter of 1796 and Kant recognized in it Hufeland's attempt to fulfill Kant's demand that the physical (and physiological) aspects of the human being be treated "morally." Kant recognized that Hufeland's argument for prophylaxis is to avoid illness, rather than using specific foods for treatment in a philosophy of moral life. He relates this to the Stoic notion of "endurance and moderation."[25]

Kant's essay (as with many of these presentations concerning diet and longevity, as we shall see in the next chapter) is highly autobiographical. His discussion of diet is tangibly tied to his awareness of his own aging body.[26] He compares himself against men in their prime and he defines aging specifically in gendered terms. He speaks of the increased amount of liquid that "aged men" seem to need to drink, which then disturbs their sleep. For Kant the power of the rational mind to avoid illness rests in the control that the mind has not only over what is ingested, but also the very control of breathing and the body. It is the will that controls the body. Part of this rationale is explained in a final footnote, in which Kant speaks of the blindness in one of his eyes and his anxiety about the failing sight in the other. He distances this fear by asking whether the pathologies of vision are in the eye or in the processing of visual data by the brain. Unlike diet, which can be manipulated to control the health (and weight) of the body, the aging body seems to have its own rate of decline for which there is no control, even in rationality. Kant's essay, which begins with Hufeland's dietetics, ends with the aging, half-blind philosopher ruminating on the irresistible but fascinating decay of his own body.

Popular philosophy too turned to obesity as a topic in the Enlightenment. Benjamin Franklin (1706–90) expressed a continuous interest in food and the particular ways in which one could eat. Franklin, while presenting himself to the readership of his widely read autobiography (published in 1791, after his death) as a man of simple tastes, most definitely enjoyed food. His later stress on simple and therefore healthy foods he credited to the simple foods he was served in the poverty of his youth in Boston. In addition to the attainment of simple tastes, Franklin's childhood taught him to consider meals and eating to be a social function. His views were self-consciously opposed to the table etiquette as well as the foodstuffs of the wealthy, both at home in Philadelphia and later in London and Paris.

At age 16, Franklin read Thomas Tyron's *The Way to Health, Long Life and Happiness* (1695), which recommended, "Temperance in eating and drinking, and moderation in their sleep and exercise. By such methods as these the seeds of vice might more easily…be subdued and a foundation laid for the building upon an excellent and accomplished person." It is the morality of good diet that appealed to Franklin. Franklin strictly followed this vegetable diet for a short while. He soon started eating fish, reasoning that, "when the Fish were opened, I saw smaller Fish taken out of their stomachs: Then thought I, if you eat one another, I don't see why we mayn't eat you."[27] The philosophy Tyron expressed in his book pervaded into Franklin's moral virtues, which he included in his writing of *Poor Richard's Almanack*. While Franklin did enjoy both eating and drinking, he tried not to overdo either one, as he stated in *Poor Richard's Almanack*, "Eat not to dullness. Drink not to elevation."[28] Also included in one of Franklin's many versions of *Poor Richard's*, was his instruction to fellow countrymen, "to supply our selves from our own Produce at home."

As an avid traveler, Franklin enjoyed tastes and recipes from abroad; yet, he still remained true to American food and flavors. In the 1742 version of his wildly popular *Poor Richard's Almanack*, the section, "Rules of Health and Long Life, and to Preserve from Malignant Fevers, and Sickness in General," demonstrates Franklin's dedication to eating for health and his ability to reduce his philosophy of life to proverbial form. Franklin was also an advocate of the strenuous life. His belief in swimming as a sport made it popular in England, where William Wyndham offered to fund Franklin's creation of the first swim club. As with diet it was a book that Franklin had read, Melchisedec Thevenot's *The Art of Swimming and Advice for Bathing* (1696), that persuaded him of the health benefits of exercise. With all of this said, and while Franklin did avidly believe in eating for health—he no doubt enjoyed his Spartan diet and engaged in healthful exercise—he was over 300 lb (21 stones 6 lb.) at the time he died.

Scientists and lay people alike from the late seventeenth to early nineteenth century began to think of the human body more and more as a machine, and then later as a collection of chemical processes. With the Enlightenment, obesity became one of the diseases that modern medicine had to confront. Obesity was no longer a sign of sin and excess, as the types and numbers of people who had sufficient access to food to become overweight increased. The middle-class world needed to see obesity as a medical (rather than a moral or social) problem and the physicians obliged. Obesity is to be overcome through medical treatment and such treatments as dieting and exercise, become the means of self-liberation, self-control, or self-limitation. They are processes by which individuals show their ability to understand their sense of social responsibility as well as their sense of responsibility to the self.

The beginning of a "modern" (i.e., materialist) science of medicine saw the development of the view that human beings proceed along an arch of development and that there is a specific moment where the body is most at risk from obesity. In 1757, the Dutch physician Malcolm Flemyng (1700–64) argued for the inheritance of a tendency toward obesity in a presentation to the Royal College of Physicians in London. His *A Discourse on the Nature, Causes, and Cures of Corpulency* (1757) argued for a physiological rather than a moral definition of obesity: fat people are not inherently lazy or sinful. His cure is exercise early on as "persons inclined to corpulency seldom think on reducing their size till they grow very bulky and then they scarce can or will use exercise enough to be remarkably serviceable." Thomas Jameson in 1811 felt that the period from the twenty-eighth to the fifty-eighth year was the height of male perfection.[29] Kant would have agreed with this. And yet this is also the age of the most danger, as "We...find corpulency steals imperceptibly on most men, between the ages of 30 and 57. In many instances the belly becomes prominent, and the person acquires a more upright gait."[30] Yet this is not necessarily a bad thing, as "A moderate degree of obesity is certainly a desirable state of body at all times, as it indicates a healthy condition of the assimilating powers..."[31] Obesity "also diminishes the irritability of the system, since fat people are remarked for good humor, and for bearing cold better that those who are lean, on account of the defensive coat of fat surrounding their nerves."[32] But fat can become dangerous: "When the heart and great vessels are so oppressed with fat, as to render the pulse slow and feeble, and the respiration difficult, the cumbrous load becomes of more serious import to the health..."[33] The "prominent belly" is "considered as the first symptom of decay, particularly as it is generally observed to continue through a great part of old age."[34] Here again the shadow of the Greek humors reappear to claim that the phlegmatic body and the aged body have the same underlying pathology, that of obesity.

In eighteenth-century Britain, the Scots physician and diet therapist George Cheyne (1672–1743) wrote his *Essay on Health and Long Life* (1724). George Cheyne's autobiography is appended not to his book on longevity but notably to his 1733 handbook, *The English Malady, or, a Treatise of Nervous Diseases of all Kinds, as Spleen, Vapours, Lowness of Spirits, Hypochondrical, and Hysterical Distempers* (London: G. Strahan, 1733). Life experience becomes the basis for his claim on the authenticity of his understanding of how to cure the obese body.

Cheyne studied medicine in Edinburgh and established himself in London by the beginning of the eighteenth century as one of the most successful (and interesting) figures on the

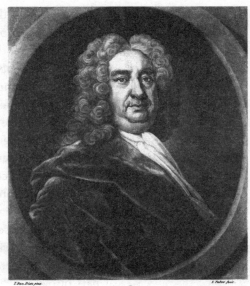

Georgius Cheynæus. M.D.
et Societatis Regiæ Socius.
Ætat: 59. 1732. *Sold at the Great Toy Shop in Bath.*

8. George
Cheyne.
Mezzotint by J.
Faber, junior, after
J. van Diest, 1732.
(Wellcome
Collection)

medical scene. Racked with self-doubt after a number of his books were either ignored or attacked, he had a massive breakdown at the age of 42. The cause of the ailments is clear in Cheyne's account. While he came from healthy parents, one side of his family was corpulent. He himself was not as a child, because he lived the life of the mind "in great Temperance."[35] His predisposition to fat, he states, is triggered when he moves to London, where he falls into the company of "Bottle-Companions, the younger Gentry, and Free-Livers."[36] The sole purpose of this companionship is to eat and drink. Taken up by them, Cheyne "grew daily in Bulk" and after a few years he grew "excessively fat, short-breathed, Lethargic, and Listless."[37]

He then began to suffer from a series of illnesses, each of which was more difficult than the last to cure. Fits followed fever. As he became more and more ill, his friends abandoned him, "leaving me to pass the melancholy Moments with my own Apprehensions and Remorse." Such friendship, founded on "sensual pleasures and mere Jollity," were false, as they were not rooted in "Virtue and in Conformity to the Divine Order."[38]

Forced to retire to the country, Cheyne began to diet, stripping his daily food down to the barest and he "melted away like a Snowball in Summer." He became a follower of the growing craze for vegetarianism, ascribing his new health to a diet of milk, fruit, roots, and seeds. In many ways he was the first celebrity "diet doc." But Cheyne also claims that this was easier for him as he had been lead astray rather than having given into the vices of London society. He was able to cure himself because he remained an outsider to the "Vices and Infidelity" that was the modern, urban world. In this, Cheyne sees society as the cause for his ailments, and the countryside and the acknowledgement of "natural Religion"[39] as the cure. Cheyne's image of the country as the refuge from a life of dissipation and the place where the obese, ill body could be reconstituted as a healthy, male body is a reflection on the newly emerging belief that the ideal state of nature is the only place where healthy, thin, and beautiful bodies exist.

Cheyne's cure was not limited to the countryside and he also attempted to be cured by waters at Bath and at Bristol.[40] He dieted, and he regularly vomited and purged—and he lost weight. And yet he continued to have illness after illness. He finally went onto a "milk diet" suggested by one of his physicians who had used it himself. No alcohol in any form, no meats, only milk, and the physician claimed that he could play six hours of cricket without tiring. Cheyne reduced his meat and alcohol intake, adding vegetables, seeds, bread, "mealy roots, and fruit."[41] The weight continued to come off. He became "Lank, Fleet, and Nimble."[42] Riding ten to fifteen miles a day, he felt he was fit even though he continued to purge and vomit. He suddenly felt that he could add some meat, chicken, and a few stronger liquors. He also stopped exercising and soon became very ill again. He then returned to his diet for twenty years and continued "sober, moderate, and plain."[43] And yet, over time, this sober and moderate diet came to add more and more foods, alcohol, meat, and nuts. See-saw dieting is not an invention of the twentieth century; nor is cheating on a diet plan. Cheyne's weight returned and he again became "enormous": "I was ready to faint away, for want to Breath, and my Face turn'd Black." Upon trying to walk up a flight of stairs he was "seiz'd with a Convulsive Asthma."[44] His body was covered in ulcers and he began to suffer from gout. The pain forced him back on his milk diet. All along he suffered from "Sickness, Retching, Lowness, Watchfullness, Eructation, and Melancholy."[45] His mental state was as bad as his physical one.

Yet all along he continued to practice as a physician: "I attended indeed (in a manner) the Business of my profession, and took Air and Exercise regularly in the Daytime; but in such a wretched, dying Condition as was evident to all that saw me."[46] He was persuaded to return to London at the end of 1725, where he then met with his medical friends, who were not the dandies that had abandoned him. He tried to return to the earlier diet but was suddenly aware that the flexibility of youth had diminished and that he had to be ever more watchful and vigilant in his present state.[47] This meant no meat, little alcohol, and a modicum of medicinal Port. In the end, Cheyne believed that obese individuals could only be brought around to a healthy diet: "no one will ever be brought to such a Regimen as mine is now, without having been first extremely Miserable; and I think Common Life, with temperance, is best for the Generality, else it would not be Common."[48]

What Cheyne ate is familiar to us from Cornaro: "The Simplicity of the Alimentary Gospel." He avoided "onions and garlic."[49] Still, he continued to suffer from flatulence and eruction—belching—for a time. But he became fit, able to "be abroad in all Weathers, Seasons or Times of the Year, day or Night, without much Dread or Hazard of Cold."[50] More importantly, when he had a carriage accident and was knocked unconscious, he was able to recover, according to him, because of the new state of his health.[51] Dieting preserves life in all cases and makes one a better and more moral human being. Cheyne's powerful view that only vegetarianism furthers the sensitive nature of man became part of the image of the vegetarian. Jean-Jacques Rousseau was to argue, using a Cheynian view, that the English were "cruel and ferocious" because of the "roast beef."

But the merger between medicine and religion should not be underestimated even in the age of a radical medical rationalism. John Wesley (1703–91), founder of Methodism and the author of what was one of the best selling popular medical handbooks in England from 1750–1850, noted in 1747 that, "Nothing conduces more to health, than abstinence and plain food with due labour. For studious persons, about eight ounces of animal food, and twelve of vegetable in twenty-four hours is sufficient."[52] Diet is central, yet, "A due degree of exercise is indispensably necessary to health and long life."[53]

Wesley's view on diet owed much to his reading of the dietary physician Cheyne as a student at Oxford. His dietetics argued appropriateness of food and quantities for good health. One must "suit the quality and quantity of the food to the strength of our digestion; to take always such a sort and such a measure of food as fits light and easy to the stomach." But his views also reflected his own theological acceptance of fasting as part of a rejection of the sumptuous foods of modern life. For him, fasting becomes a divinely inspired means by which the individual and the community acknowledge the need for abstemious self-denial to praise God, expiate sin, and avert divine wrath. To this he added the benefits to health of fasting, which he borrows from Cheyne's dietetics. For Wesley, fasting is a form of dieting to cure the results of the sin of the "excess of food...they have indulged in their sensual appetites, perhaps even impairing their bodily health, certainly to the no small hurt of their soul." Fasting is thus the abstention "from what had well nigh plunged them in everlasting perdition. They often wholly refrain; always take care to be sparing and temperate in all things." Health is not merely a divine state but it is the absence of the sin of gluttony. It can be achieved through dieting.[54]

From Alvise Luigi Cornaro's Renaissance Venice to John Wesley's London we can see an effortless merger of religion and science in the Enlightenment, an age seemingly dedicated, if we are to believe Voltaire, to the exile of superstition from the age of rationalism. Religion and science remain connected in the realm of obesity as a category that reflects both moral and somatic causes. We have moved, however, from food as therapy to food as danger. Obesity remains a conflicted focus of all of the discussions of the nature of illness and of the relationship of the body to the divine.

IV

THE BATTLE BETWEEN SCIENCE AND MORALITY FOR THE CURE OF OBESITY

Religion and science continued to debate the nature and meaning of obesity well past the Enlightenment. Given the fact that these two aspects of the public sphere continue to be seen in the twenty-first century as the warfare between "theology" and "science" (the title of a major book of 1896 by the historian of science Andrew Dickson White) the debate seems have been stuck in the "which is right" or the "apologetics" mode. The history of obesity shows that religion appropriated the arguments of a new science to provide rationales and explanations for the nature of obesity. There have been debates, for and against, about the healthy nature of food *within* religious practices in the West since the nineteenth century, and they continue today. Religion appropriated the findings of health science ("hygiene") and the meaning of the healthy body as the "Temple of God" very early on. Not the warfare between "theology" and "science" but its public integration is central to the history of obesity. Somatic as well as psychological explanations found in science come to affect religious understanding of obesity as a sign of the unhealthy body.

By the end of the eighteenth century, a new idea enters the understanding of the cause and the treatment of the obese, the failure of mind rather than the failure of the body. "Gula" is given a psychological rather than a moral meaning. Such views of the "will" and its diseases were first formulated in the nineteenth century when psychology turned obesity and extreme thinness into a truly voluntary act in which (according to the psychologist Thomas Reid [1710–96]) "Every man is conscious of a power to determine, in things which he conceives of to depend upon his determination."[1] This faculty could become ill, resulting in pathologies of the will. The major psychiatrists wrote of this, from J. E. D. Esquirol (1772–1840) to Théodule Ribot (1839–1916) in his *The Diseases of the Will* (1884) and Henry Maudsley (1835–1918) in his *Body and Mind: An Inquiry Into Their Connection and Mutual Influence* (1870). The psychiatric diagnosis that resulted was "aboulia," the inability to execute what one wants to do, without any sign of physical impairment. In this, there is no ability to move from motive and desire to execution.

The idea that a weakness of will was the cause of obesity became a medical as well as a popular trope by the end of the eighteenth century. "Obesity," as the French writer on taste Jean Anthelme Brillat-Savarin (1755–1826) states in *The Physiology of Taste or, Meditations on Transcendental Gastronomy* (1825), his handbook on food and diet at the beginning of the nineteenth century, "is not actually a disease, it is at least a most unpleasant state of ill health, and one into which we almost always fall because of our own fault."[2] Obesity comes to be the stuff of popular concern. Samuel Johnson defined obesity in his *Dictionary of the English Language* (1755) as "loaden with flesh", and did define diet both in the older sense of "food, provisions

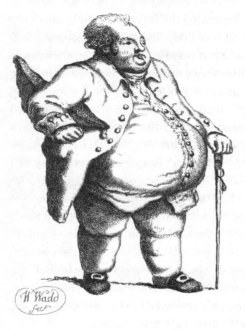

Frontispiece.

Comments on Corpulency.

Published by John Ebers & Cᵒ London 1829.

9. A large gentleman with a walking stick. From William Wadd, *Comments on Corpulency. Lineaments of Leanness. Mems on Diet and Dietetics* (London: John Ebers & Co., 1829). (Wellcome Collection)

for the mouth; victuals" as well as the more modern sense of "food regulated by the rules of medicine, for the prevention or cure of any disease." ("Obesity" was introduced into English in the seventeenth century as a popular medical term equivalent to the Latin medical term *adipose*. It appears as early as

Thomas Blount's dictionary *Glossographia* of 1661.) Johnson, whose body was then racked by innumerable ailments, both inherited and acquired, undertook such a "cure" in September of 1780: "I am now beginning the seventy-second year of my life, with more strength of body and greater vigour of mind than, I think, is common at that age ... I have been attentive to my diet, and have diminished the bulk of my body."[3]

James Boswell's (1740–95) biography, *The Life of Samuel Johnson LLD* (1791), noted that Johnson (1709–84) viewed obesity as purely a product of bad diet: "whatever be the quantity that a man eats, it is plain that if he is too fat, he has eaten more that he should have done."[4] Boswell, however, disagreed with Johnson, stating, "You will see one man fat who eats moderately, and another lean who eats a great deal."[5] This was in response to Johnson, who said that he "fasted from the Sunday's dinner to the Tuesday's dinner, without any inconvenience."[6] Boswell noted that this may well have been true, but he also explained that Johnson could "practise abstinence, but not temperance."[7] This means of understanding obesity as a psychological weakness is quickly answered by the new science of the body, which defines it solely as a somatic ailment.

The first of the modern exponents of a "scientific" diet rather than a moral or psychological treatment for obesity was William Banting, (1796–1878), an English undertaker. (There were other celebrated gurus of weight reduction before Banting, such as William Wood [1719–83], who advocated following the teachings of Cornaro, but Banting was the first true "celebrity dieter.") His *Letter on Corpulence Addressed to the Public* was an account of how a successful, middle class undertaker and coffin maker (he had actually supplied the coffin for the Duke of Wellington) overcame his fat. He was not fat because

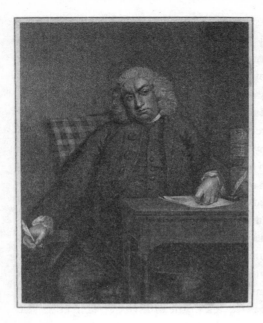

10. Samuel
Johnson. From
James Boswell, *The
Life of Samuel
Johnson LLD*
(London: Cadell
and Davies, 1816).
(*Wellcome
Collection*)

of inaction or lassitude: "Few men have led a more active life—
bodily or mentally—from a constitutional anxiety for regularity,
precision, and order, during fifty years' business career...so
that my corpulence and subsequent obesity was not through
neglect of necessary bodily activity, nor from excessive eating,
drinking, or self-indulgence of any kind."[8] And yet, at the age of
66, he stood at about 5 feet 5 inches tall and weighed 202 pounds
(14 stones 6 lb.). He sensed that he had stopped being corpulent
and had become obese. A "corpulent man eats, drinks, and
sleeps well, has no pain to complain of, and no particular
organic disease."[9] But obesity was now understood as the
source of specific illnesses. He developed "obnoxious boils,"[10]
failing sight and hearing, and a "slight umbilical rupture."[11]

62

He could neither stoop to tie his shoes "nor attend to the little offices humanity requires without considerable pain and difficulty."[12] Indeed, he was "compelled to go down stairs slowly backward."[13] All of these pathologies were seen by Banting (and his physicians agreed) as the direct result of his obesity rather than his aging. In the appendix to the second edition, still distributed for free, Banting states that "I am told by all who know me that my personal appearance is greatly improved, and that I seem to bear the stamp of good health; this may be a matter of opinion or a friendly remark, but I can honestly assert that I feel restored in health, 'bodily and mentally,' appear to have more muscular power and vigour, eat and drink with a good appetite, and sleep well."[14] Health is beauty.

Most galling for Banting, however, was the social stigma: "No man labouring under obesity can be quite insensible to the sneers and remarks of the cruel and injudicious in public assemblies, public vehicles, or the ordinary street traffic... He naturally keeps away as much as possible from places where he is likely to be made the object of the taunts and remarks of others."[15] Underlying Banting's desire to lose weight is the fact that he was seen as a fat man and his body was perceived as useless and parasitic. Stigma, as much as physical disability, accounted for Banting's sense of his own illness.

Having been unable to achieve weight loss through the intervention of physicians, Banting was desperate. One physician urged him to exercise and he rowed daily, which gave him only a great appetite. Another physician told him that weight gain was a natural result of aging and that he had gained a pound for every year since he had attained manhood.[16] Indeed, the medical literature of the mid-nineteenth century had come to consider obesity a problem of medical therapy; it condemned self-help: "Domestic medicine is fraught with innumerable evils—it is false economy to practice physic upon yourselves, when a little judicious guidance would obviate all difficulties."[17] He took the waters at Leamington, Cheltenham, and Harrogate; he took Turkish baths at a rate of up to three a week for a year but lost only six pounds in all that time, and had less and less energy. Nothing helped.

Failing to find a treatment for his weakened hearing, he turned to William Harvey, an ear, nose and throat specialist and a Fellow of the Royal College of Surgeons in August 1862. Harvey had heard Claude Bernard lecture in Paris on the role that the liver had in diabetes.[18] Bernard believed that in addition to secreting bile, the liver also secreted something that aided in the metabolism of sugars. Harvey began to examine the role that the various types of foods, specifically starches and sugars, had in diseases such as diabetes. He urged Banting to reduce the amount of these in his diet, for, he argued, "that certain articles of ordinary diet, however beneficial in youth, are prejudicial in advanced life, like beans to a horse, whose common food is hay and corn."[19] The aging body could not use the common diet and needed much less sugar and starch.

Such an approach is hardly unique: for Jean Anthelme Brillat-Savarin in 1825 the reduction of "grains and starches" must be at the center of any weight-loss diet.[20] The fat man objects: "Here in a single word he forbids us everything we most love, those little white rolls from Limet, and Archard's cakes, and those cookies from...". Yet Brillat-Savarin is adamant: "Shun anything made with flour..., you still have the roast, the salad, the leafy vegetables."[21]

With this new approach Banting's body finally began to shed its excess weight. He lost 35 lb., could walk down stairs "naturally," take ordinary exercise, and could "perform every necessary office for himself," his rupture was better, and he could hear and see.[22] But equally important, his "dietary table was far superior to the former—more luxurious and liberal, independent of its blessed effect."[23] He remained at a normal weight until his death in London in 1878 at the age of 81. Not quite a hundred, but not bad either.

Banting's pamphlet became a best-seller and started a serious, scientific concern as to the meaning of obesity. It was actually one of a number of such pamphlets of the day. One, by A. W. Moore in 1857, cited Cornaro as the prime case of one who was able to loss weight and become healthy.[24] Watson Bradshaw, a physician who had written on dyspepsia before Banting's pamphlet appeared, countered it in 1864 with his own work on obesity warning against "rash experiment upon themselves in furtherance of that object." For Watson Bradshaw, the ideal of the fat body in cultures such as China and Turkey where the "*ultima thule* of human beauty is to possess a face with a triple chin, and a huge abdomen" had become impossible in the West.[25] It was impossible because the "assimilative function has changed its character—the absorbents have varied their duties—fat forsakes the lower extremities and other parts of the body; and persists in concentrating itself in the abdomen, giving rise to what is called 'Corpulence.'"[26] Corpulence is a condition of the modern, Western age, and concentrated as it is in the gut, a quality of men. It is clear that this is a pathological state for Bradshaw, but it is the only extreme cases that he sees as diseased. In a pamphlet of 1865, "A London Physician" wrote about "How to Get Fat or the Means of Preserving the Medium Between Leanness and Obesity."[27] He begins by saying that the one question that everyone asks is, "Have you read Banting?" and this has "invaded all classes, and doubtless, will descend to posterity."[28] He explains that: "Corpulence is a parasite, that the parasite is a disease, and the close ally of a disease, and the said parasite has been exposed and his very existence threatened" by writers such as Banting and William Harvey. This pamphlet then turned to the emaciated body, which is seen as equally at risk and in need of diet and reform.

But it was Banting's text that became most popular because it was sold as autobiographical. People spoke of "banting" when they tried to shed weight. Even today, Swedish term for "dieting" is "*bantning*." The obese patient was the subject of reform, and for a rather long time, the patient was seen as a European one. Banting's mentor, William Harvey, turned to this topic in 1872, spurred on, he wrote, by Banting's success. Harvey stressed that the new scientific advances in "physiology and animal chemistry"[29] have meant that one could treat obesity as a disease. He quotes Banting as an authority. Suddenly, sufferer and physician saw obesity as the product of forces beyond the will. But Harvey agreed with Banting that until this stage of pathology is reached, "persons rarely become objects of attention; many have even congratulated themselves on their comely appearance, not seeking advice or a remedy for that which they did not consider an evil..."[30] One of Banting's severest contemporary critics, the Scots physician William E. Aytoun, observed that: "We are acquainted with many estimable persons of both sexes, turning considerably more than fifteen stone in the scales—a heavier weight than Mr. Banting ever attained—whose health is unexceptionable, and who would laugh to scorn the idea of applying to a doctor for recipe or regimen which might have the effect of marring their developed comeliness."[31]

Banting and Harvey redefined obesity as a physiological disease rather than as a fashion or a moral failing. Yet Harvey could not make a sufficient leap between his knowledge and the actual mechanism by which "respiratory foods" (carbohydrates) caused obesity and then other ailments. It was Felix Niemeyer from Stuttgart who later argued that it was the ingestion of more or less pure protein that would reduce the toxic effects of sugars and starches. All believed that the body was a collection of chemical processes. Questions of will and its attendant diseases were eliminated.

One advocate of modern, scientific interventions for obesity was John Henry Kellogg, M.D. (1852–1943), who employed a wide range of cutting-edge treatments at the Battle Creek Sanitarium. While today best known for his invention of flaked breakfast cereals, Kellogg was also one of the most outspoken health reformers dealing with obesity in the late nineteenth century. Raised as a Seventh-day Adventist, he was inspired by founder Ellen G. White's (1827–1915), writings on health reform, which stressed healthy living as a religious duty. Here again religious belief and obesity come into close proximity as science is taken up in the service of religious belief.

After the Great Disappointment of October 22, 1844, when Christ failed to return as predicted by the Millerite sect of Christianity, Ellen G. White reorganized a movement based on visions that she claimed had been sent by God to her during trances.

As part of her reconstruction of a Sabbatarian dietary code, she propagated a dietary philosophy aimed at cultivating and preparing Christian souls for the second coming. "I was informed that the inhabitants of earth had been degenerating, losing their strength and comeliness. Satan has the power of disease and death, and with every age the effects of the curse have been more visible and the power of Satan more plainly seen."[32] In 1864, her husband Rev. James White became ill, and White nursed him back to health using rigorous vegetarian principles. In 1866 they founded the Western Health Reform Institute at Battle Creek, Michigan, which became the center for late-nineteenth-century diet reform. White sees the Garden of Eden as the model for the modern diet: "God gave our first parents the food He designed that the race should eat. It was contrary to His plan to have the life of any creature taken. There was to be no death in Eden. The fruit of the trees in the garden was the food man's wants required," she wrote in 1864.[33]

Sexual reform was also part of the practice of hygiene in Battle Creek. White was a stern critic of the "solitary vice," masturbation. She preached against a variety of foods and other commodities such as meat, alcohol, tobacco, and spices, which she believed excited the nervous system and led to "self-abuse." This, in turn led to physical deformities, and even early death. In 1864, she printed a pamphlet warning against this evil, entitled *An Appeal to Mothers: The Great Cause of the Physical, Mental and Moral Ruin of Many of the Children of Our Time*.

White also preached against medical intervention in case of ill health and recommended a regimen of fresh air, sunshine, exercise, vegetarian food, and plenty of water as a cure for any ailment. She constantly linked religious conviction with notions of hygiene: "The majority of the diseases which the human family have been and still are suffering under, they have created by ignorance of their own organic health, and work perseveringly to tear themselves to pieces, and when broken down and debilitated in body and mind, send for the doctor and drug themselves to death," she wrote in 1866. Again in 1902, she warned against the diseased nature of modern food: "Flesh was never the best food; but its use is now doubly objectionable, since disease in animals is so rapidly increasing." White's teachings were characteristic of the American health reform movement's emphasis on temperance and abstemious living and shaped much of the reforms advocated by Kellogg, who clearly followed her model of therapy within allopathic medicine.

Kellogg's published works range from a monthly Adventist magazine called *Health Reformer* to an anti-tobacco book, *Tobaccoism or How Tobacco Kills* (1922), to *Plain Facts about Sexual Life* (1877). The linking of all types of reform, including sexual reform, was part of the moralizing tendency in which diet and dieting played a large role in nineteenth- and twentieth-century America.

In his *The Stomach: Its Disorders, and How to Cure Them* (1896), Kellogg presents a cure for the new "American malady," dyspepsia. For him "Americans enjoyed the unenviable, but nevertheless deserved, reputation of being a nation of dyspeptics."[34] It is dyspepsia, rather than George Miller Beard's "American disease" of "neurasthenia" (1869) that defined the pathology of modernity for Kellogg. Indeed, he lumps such nervous disorders under "gastric neurasthenia" and argues that they can be cured through diet, rather than through electrotherapy. To prove this, Kellogg presented his theory of diet and dieting in light of the newest science of bacteriology. It is a new science for a new, reformed America.

Quoting Pasteur, David, and others who showed that the digestive tract is full of "a vast number of microbes capable of producing various acids, poisonous ptomaines and toxins," he argues that only correct dieting can prevent disease.[35] It is the "modern stomach" that demands a modern cure for this "formidable disease."[36] He provides a detailed list of what to do, including slow and regular chewing[37] and the avoidance of substances like vinegar (because it is "an alcoholic liquor"),[38] too much sugar,[39] uncooked food,[40] and abundant use of fat. But most importantly, Kellogg provides a detailed diet regimen for all people to follow to prevent or to cure dyspepsia. He begins with an "aseptic dietry," which advocates sterilized food prepared without milk or eggs, whole grains, fresh fruits raw, or cooked without sugar or with grains.[41] Page upon page of proscriptive diets follows, all of which are intended to cure and prevent various forms of disease. In addition, all of Kellogg's diets adapted the idea of vegetarianism with the addition of claiming that the preparation or manufacture of the foods was now an intrinsic part of the cure of obesity. Not alone the Garden of Eden but also American manufacturing was now central to the discipline of the body.

Kellogg's dietary beliefs may have been influenced by his professional training but were also the result of a general interest in health reform at the time. Kellogg was trained as a surgeon at Bellevue Hospital Medical College in New York. Shortly after receiving his medical degree, he became superintendent of the Western Health Reform Institute in Michigan, which he renamed Battle Creek Sanitarium (also known as "The San."). The health retreat became the most popular health sanatorium of its time, boasting patients like Henry Ford (1863–1947), John D. Rockefeller (1839–1947), and J.C. Penney (1875–1971). Patients at "the San." closely followed Kellogg's "Battle Creek Idea," a diet that excluded meat, and recommended sparing use of eggs, refined sugar, milk, and cheese.

This demanded a "lifestyle change," which advocated abstaining from alcohol, tea, coffee, tobacco, and chocolate. The diet also prescribed daily enemas, drinking large quantities of water, and participating in regular exercise and outdoor activity.

"The San." was originally affiliated with the Adventist Church but had moved away from religious practice to a more medical and scientific focus by 1907. Kellogg now appealed to "rational medicine" as, "Nature alone possesses the power to heal." As in "The San.," "patients, and not disease are to be treated."[42] As such, "The San." included a "Laboratory of Hygiene" that aimed to create new nutritious food products by undertaking the "preliminary digestive work" of the body by "kettle cooking, oven cooking, and toasting."[43]

Kellogg's brother, William Keith Kellogg (1860–1951), joined him in his research, and they began experimenting with new kinds of grain products, imitation meats, coffee substitutes, and soya milk. At this time, manufactured and processed foods were believed to be healthier than "natural" foods. In 1895, they accidentally left a batch of boiled grain (dough) out for several days, allowing it to dry out and become crisp. When they rolled out the dried dough, it formed flakes and a new kind of cereal was born. The flakes, originally named Granose and later known as Toasted Wheat Flakes, immediately became popular, and they sold over 100,000 pounds of the cereal in the first year. The Kellogg brothers established Sanitas Food Company for their new products but experienced major ideological differences relating to both health reform and business. The company split into John's Battle Creek Food Company and William's W. K. Kellogg Company. The latter went on to become one of the most popular food companies, ironically abandoning the "health food" label of its origins. Many have argued today that it was the advent of convenience food that led to many of the problems with obesity, currently considered a major public health problem in the modern world.

Kellogg was inspired by the American Presbyterian minister, social reformer, and early advocate of dietary reform Sylvester Graham (1794–1851). Graham was chronically ill as a young man, diagnosed with "consumption" (tuberculosis), which interrupted his studies at Amherst College. After one of his illnesses, he married his nurse. As a preacher he was an advocate of the "temperance" movement. In 1830, while preaching in Pennsylvania against the dangers of drink, he met members of the Vegetarian Bible Christian Church and thereafter became an advocate of vegetarianism. After 1839 he withdrew from his public activities to devote himself to developing his system. Like many reformers of his day, Graham associated capitalism with moral decay. Responding in part to the advent of pre-prepared foods, Graham wrote his famous *Treatise on Bread, and Bread-Making* (1837), in which he urged readers to make quality bread at home and eat it fresh. His Graham bread was made primarily with wholewheat and molasses, as opposed to white flour, and it contained neither yeast nor eggs. The ideal food came to be bread. It was plain, unadorned, and true to itself. As Catharine Beecher was to write a decade later of "Nourishing and Unstimulating Food," that "wheat stands at the head, as the most nutritive, safe, and acceptable diet to all classes and in all circumstances. This can be used in the form of bread, every day, through a whole life, without cloying the appetite, and to an extent that can be said of no other food."[44] Graham was also a staunch advocate of vegetarianism, and apparently the first American to link a philosophy of vegetarianism to a physiological argument about health. Others of his time shared his belief that to kill animals was barbaric and that a vegetarian diet reinforced better elements of human nature, but for Graham it was also medicalized, as he believed vegetarian diets led to longer life.

Graham's advocacy of a pure diet was very much linked to sexual reform. In his 1834 *Lecture to Young Men on Chastity* his motto is, "Beware the fleshly lusts, which war against the soul."[45] Human beings, he notes, have "two grand functions… that are necessary for [their] existence…The first is *nutrition*; the second is *reproduction*."[46] He condemns "self-pollution" as more dangerous even than the "illicit commerce between the sexes"[47] as it "ruins the physical constitution."[48] Sex should be treated as he imagines food must be: "when we eat and drink for the purpose of sustaining our bodies in the best condition with the ulterior view of promoting the healthiest and most vigorous state of our intellectual faculties…"[49] rather than merely "pandering to our appetites." It is the stomach that "more directly and powerfully fully sympathizes with the genital organs, in all their excitement and affections, than any other organ or portion of the body."[50] Bread and pure foods would cure the ravages of masturbation as well as dampen sexual excess. The moral question became a question of the control of the body through specific foods. His eccentric diet prohibited consumption not only of meat, but also of tea, alcohol, spices, and sweets because of their intensifying effects on the sexual drives of men, women, and children alike. For Graham, diet was essential. Without dietary reform no reform or rehabilitation was possible.

In his *Lectures on the Science of Human Life* (1839) Graham argued for a Divine self-awareness of man that led him first to eat of the fruits surrounding him.[51] He rejects the argument of the scientists of his day, such as Georges-Louis Leclerc, Comte de Buffon (1707–88), that man is an omnivorous animal. For Graham, the very anatomy of the human being predisposes him to eat fruits and vegetables. Man is a herbivorous animal, whose teeth and digestive system are predisposed not to eat meat. He rejects, therefore, the common notion of the day that "Animal food renders man strong and courageous," while a vegetable diet is "...connected with weakness and cowardice."[52] The best of human society in history subsisted on vegetables and fruits—from the Spartans to the Romans—while "Natural Man," such as those ranked as on the lowest rung of humanity of the day, the inhabitants of Terra del Fuego in Argentina, eat 15 to 20 pounds of barely cooked flesh a day, which leads to their "indolence."[53] Modern man must be healthy and able to work; this is possible only through a meatless diet.

Graham, White, and Kellogg had numerous disciples, who moved religious attitudes toward obesity into the world of commerce. Perhaps the best known of these is Charles William Post (1854–1914) who built the Postum Cereal Company as one of the major players in the American food reform movement of the late nineteenth century and, incidentally, made a $17 million fortune. In 1890, Post, a self-taught inventor and salesman, arrived at John Harvey Kellogg's Battle Creek Sanitarium in Michigan because of his own failing health. During his visit, Post became exposed to the food reform movement and its claims about human health. Here he experienced the use of breakfast cereals as the basis for health therapies, using the double idea of a "modern" health regime with a "religious" foundation.

Here, Post, like all of the cereal manufacturers of the time, followed the lead of Henry Perky (1843–1906) who had developed the "wheat shredding process" and created shredded wheat. Post called on "science" with his advocacy of a "true domestic science" that "should be taught in all our schools,"[54] but he also condemned American Protestantism with its lack of a strict dietary regime as one of the causes of American ill health. In contrast, he praised the strict regime of Judaism and Islam for their attention to diet.[55] All aimed toward bodily control including that of the obese body.

Post left the sanitarium after nine months and purchased a farm in Battle Creek, where he began experimenting with grain-based health foods and beverages, which he was introduced to at Kellogg's sanitarium but found almost uneatable due to the bland taste. Post then founded La Vita Inn at Battle Creek where obesity was also treated. He also advocated a mind-cure for bodily illness in his tractate *I am Well! The Modern Practice of Natural Suggestion as Distinct from Hypnotic Unnatural Influence* (1895), thus positioning himself in the "New Thought" movement dominated by figures like William James and Mary Baker Eddy, who argued, "*Disease is entirely a mental picture.*"[56] His views echoed the Social Darwinism of his day, seeing such health advocacy as improving the "race." But underlying all was the need to accommodate everything to the selling of a notion of health. In 1908 he explained, "I studied psychology, dietetics, hygiene, and medicine in this country and Europe. I have been through psychology from the book by Mrs. Eddy to the clinics of Charcot in mental therapeutics at Paris. What we say in our advertizing is a popular expression of things I believe to be vitally important to many others."[57]

By 1895, Post abandoned his foray into mental healing and planned to create an alternative to coffee and tea, and to develop a ready-made breakfast cereal that would be enjoyable and affordable as well as a treatment for unhealthy, obese bodies. His model here was clearly Kellogg and the Seventh-day Adventist vegetarian diet, but unlike them he rejected a "theological" rationale for the power of his food to heal. This was the triumph of science in the warfare between "theology" and "science." His food was seen as "modern" as it incorporated arguments about science and evolution in is claims for cure. Post developed and produced his first product, Postum cereal beverage, a caffeine-free coffee substitute. "If Coffee Don' Agree, try Postum," stated the ads. They also pictured, "The coffee fiend saved at the last gasp by changing to Postum."[58]

In 1897, Post developed Grape-Nuts, the first cold cereal, and, in 1899, he created a brand of cornflakes, to compete with Kellogg's Corn Flakes®. When he brought his version to the market he called it "Elijah's Manna," only changing the name in 1908 to Post Toasties. The outrage by ministers across the country at the appropriation of the biblical name by someone who had little interest beyond marketing caused the change. The Kellogg cereal had been developed by Will Keith Kellogg (1869–1951), who was employed by his older brother at the Sanatorium, as an attempt to bring health food to the masses. He received a patent for a corn flaking process in 1895. In 1906, W. K. Kellogg was excommunicated by the Seventh-day Adventist Church for adding sugar to his cornflakes in violation of the Church's dietary principles. Sugar and obesity were also twinned in the medical world. Post had no such principles.

Post's advertizing and marketing were his genius, and yet he too made distinct gestures to the religious culture of Battle Creek. By 1900, Battle Creek was the center of cereal production, but Post and Kellogg dominated the field. Post promoted his products by creating appealing phrases in language he believed appealed to the working class. He demanded that his salesmen "must use plain words, homely illustrations and more or less of the vocabulary of the customer...In other words talk to your customer in a way that he will instantly grasp what you have to say, and believe it." (1905)[59] As a leader of the National Association of Manufacturers, however, Post took a hard, anti-Labor line in his conflicts with Samuel Gompers, the Labor leader. Labor advocates were, according to him, "mongrels, prostitutes, and the most poisonous enemies of the common people."[60]

Post committed suicide in 1914, and within days the alternative physician E. H. Pratt at a convention of the Illinois Eclectic Medical Society had interpreted his death as the result of "intestinal problems."[61] Post might well have agreed with an explanation of mental illness resting on poor food and digestive disorders. Perhaps his life would have been saved had he only stuck to Postum and Grape-Nuts.

In modern day America, dieting culture is still articulated through a protestant Christian idiom and lexicon so that fitness culture now bears the characteristics of a religious movement.[62] Contemporary diet and fitness jargon is glutted with religious metaphors, conversion narratives, and testimonials. A corollary to this is seen in the medical field, where eating disorders are often diagnosed as a "spiritual crisis." In today's culture, marketers have profited greatly by combining two things that sell, *diet* and *religion*. The emergence of many religion-based diets has become quite popular, some of these including: the *Maker's Diet*, the *Body by God Plan*, the *What would Jesus Eat Program*, and the *Hallelujah Diet*. The dieting regimen with prayer is exemplified in books such as Deborah Pierce's *I Prayed Myself Slim* and Charlie Shedd's *Pray Your Weight Away*. The concept of sin in these books is associated with gluttony and unattractiveness. Prayer is a means by which the desired result of attractiveness can be achieved; in doing so one can be taken away from gluttony and ill health and be brought closer to God. This is an indication that sin and guilt has become a gage of fat.

Evidence of the relationship between religion and dieting is also present in support groups like Overeaters Anonymous (OA), which is a non-profit organization, originally founded to help those who suffer from compulsive eating, but now includes anorexics and bulimics, as well as compulsive eaters. The structure and philosophy of OA was based on the model of Alcoholics Anonymous (AA). Founded in 1935, AA uses a "twelve-step" program for "recovery from alcoholism." This social movement has had a considerable impact on therapy across all levels of society. Central to its message, rooted in the Judeo-Christian tradition, is the need for a particular relationship between God and oneself. The religious dimension of AA was evident enough that the "Secular Organization for Sobriety" (also known as "Save our Selves") was created as an answer. Overeaters Anonymous mirrors AA in that it claims that compulsive eating is an "emotional and spiritual disease" and is "progressive and incurable," unless one turns individual control over to God, the higher power, and asks for his help in re-evaluating life.

It is not just the religion-based therapies for obesity, however, that emphasize the need for spiritual purpose in dieting. Indeed, many contemporary dieting books suggest that either dieters need to find peace to achieve dieting success or that the diet purposed will actually bring the reader peace. From wherever the peace originates, modern science has shown that religion can be a powerful factor in dietary success. One of the reasons suggested by researchers is that the church group can be a good support system for someone looking to improve his or her health. In addition, the Sunday morning service can be a good platform to distribute information on dietary changes for healthy weight maintenance. Therefore, some investigators have used people who attend church as research subjects to test dietary interventions.

In contrast to the use of diet as a representation of austerity and reverence to God in the time of Sylvester Graham, dieting in contemporary society has a very different relationship with religion. From the use of church groups as support groups for those coping with diabetes to the Overeaters Anonymous model based on curing the spirit, dieting is intrinsically linked to a higher power in many diets.

V

A SOMATIC *OR* A PSYCHOLOGICAL TREATMENT OF OBESITY

The nineteenth century was clearly a time when religious advocates of "moral" and "healthy" food saw them as a means of combating obesity. It was also a time of radical innovations and discoveries in allopathic medicine. In 1855, the Parisian physiologist Claude Bernard (1813–78) had reshaped human biology as an experimental science. One of his experiments showed that there were "internal secretions" (hormones) from the glands that had a regulating effect on bodily systems such as digestion and metabolism. A new science of obesity developed during this new age of experimental biology and its applications to obesity. The studies of Wilbur Olin Atwater (1844–1907), an American agricultural chemist, on respiration and metabolism contributed greatly to the science of human nutrition and the problem of obesity. After receiving his PhD from Yale in 1869, for studying the chemical composition of corn, Atwater studied with German chemists and physiologists such as Nathan Zuntz (1847–1920), who developed the first portable apparatus to measure metabolism; Carl von Voit (1831–1908), who established the study of the physiology of metabolism in mammals, and his student,

Max Rubner (1854–1932), who proved that the energy released by food was the same if digested or burnt. When Atwater returned to the United States, he directed extensive studies on food analysis, dietary evaluations, energy requirements for work, digestibility of foods, and the economics of food production. The chemist Francis Gano Benedict (1870–1957) took courses from chemist Josiah Parsons Cooke (1827–1894) at Harvard, who, in 1850, founded the Harvard chemistry department. After completing his graduate study at Heidelberg University in Germany, Benedict returned to the United States to work with Wilbur Olin Atwater. Following his work with Atwater in chemistry and nutrition, Benedict also became involved with the problems of physiology and human weight. The two scientists began studies of metabolism in humans, using a respiration calorimeter, which had been created by Benedict to measure oxygen consumption and heat in the body. The machine was able to measure exact measurements of heat production and loss in animals and humans. Benedict published his results in his *An Experimental Inquiry Regarding the Nutritive Value of Alcohol*. In 1907, after the publishing of his findings, Benedict was appointed director of the newly established Carnegie Nutrition Laboratory in Boston. At the laboratory, Benedict developed new equipment, including a smaller instrument for measuring oxygen consumption in humans. Using the machine, Benedict, and fellow colleagues, studied the production of heat, changing the conditions of working, exercising, and eating or fasting on his subjects. From these studies, Benedict determined a basal metabolism in humans, and then wrote (with James Arthur Harris [1880–1930]) *A Biometric Study of Basal Metabolism in Man* (1919), which remains a classic in the field.

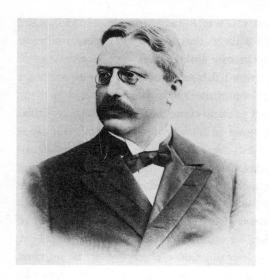

11. Carl von
Noorden. From:
Anton Mansch,
Medical World
(Berlin: Adolf
Eckstein, 1906).
(*Wellcome
Collection*)

Such figures came to embody a new scientific approach to
human weight and some figures in the treatment of pathological weight and its diseases such as the German endocrinolo-
gist, Carl von Noorden (1858–1944), became celebrity doctors
in turn-of-the-century society. Von Noorden's clinical reputation rested on the development of dietetic treatments for
diabetes and obesity. He was trained in Leipzig (obtaining his
MD in 1881) and in 1894, became Director for Internal Medicine at the City Hospital in Frankfurt am Main, where he
created a private clinic for diabetes and dietetic cures. In 1906,
he became the head of the Clinic for Internal Medicine in Imperial Vienna. In 1913, he returned to Frankfurt and then, in 1929,
returned again to Vienna (now the capital of a Republic), called
back by the new Socialist Minister of Health, Julius Tandler, as
Head of the Clinic for Metabolic Diseases. His clinical reputation rested on the development of dietetic treatments for

diabetes and obesity. It was, in fact, his understanding of the impact of diet on diabetes that shaped his understanding of obesity. He conceptually linked these two expressions of human metabolism, which is reflected in his view of the nature of obesity and the importance of a medically supervised diet.

One of Noorden's central contributions was his categorization of different types of obesity into exogenous obesity—caused by manifest overeating with less expenditure of energy—and endogenous obesity—caused by abnormalities within the body, such as faulty endocrine function.[1] Examples of an endocrine factor causing obesity are castration and hypothyroidism. Yet at the core of Noorden's movement to medicalize obesity by creating classifications for its origins was the desire to reclaim this ever-expanding category of patient from the "quacks": "reduction cures have become so popular that many patients undergo a course of treatment . . . on their own accord and without consulting a physician."[2] The legacy of William Banting was clear: self-cure meant not only fewer patients but also, more importantly, abdicating an entire arena of medicine to the quacks.

The demographics of this self-treating patient population at the turn of the century were also clear to him. Self-treatment is found more frequently in women than in men and "more commonly in young girls and in middle-aged women than in older women."[3] Among men, Noorden found that patients came to him for the treatment of symptoms, which he understood as the result of their obesity but "they do not understand how a reduction cure can be of any benefit nor how their trouble can be relieved by causing a loss of fat. . ."[4] In their own estimation, his patients were not fat and, even if they were, it had nothing to do with their complaints!

Noorden's view about the efficacy of specific diets is vague; in fact, it was clear to him that any number of diets suggested by physicians might well work. But if "the character and morals of the patient seem to indicate that they will not exercise in moderation in work and are apt to overindulge in the good things of life" the patients should be forced onto a supervised diet and sent to a sanitarium, even if there were no overt symptoms.[5] Simply sending these people for the "water cure" to reduce their weight would be useless.[6] Only medically supervised weight reduction, Noorden believed, could have the desired impact on long-term health. (Later in 1912 the doctors at the Carlsbad Baths tried unsuccessfully to get revenge by opposing his receiving the title of "Hofrat" from the Austrian Emperor.)

Noorden was very much attuned to the gender politics of his age. Thus, he advocates being very careful with "the whims and fancies of our lady patients" who, having given birth, are appalled at their abdominal fat. Radical reduction of such fat may lead, Noorden warns, to further medical complications even if changes of appearance are achieved.[7] In pathological cases, the general tendency toward a weakness of will in the obese is manifest. Hysterics (who are primarily women) "are usually persons who 'cannot' or 'will not,' whose will power is small. Subjects of this kind usually eat a great deal and are at the same time lazy so that they do not get enough muscular exercise and do not develop any energy and readily grow moderately fat."[8] Noorden placed his reduction cures in the service of a new medical science that seemed also to be answering S. Wier Mitchell's (1826–1914) "rest cure" with its goal of weight gain and enforced bed rest to "cure" neurasthenia. (Mitchell's most famous patient was Charlotte Perkins Gilman, whose short story *The Yellow Wallpaper* [1892] captures the negative psychological impact of this method.) Noorden's views impacted the later focus of obesity studies, which went on to examine factors that may regulate appetite and food consumption, such as caloric intake.

Much of Noorden's work also focused on diabetes, a disease that seemed to be increasing in late-nineteenth-century Europe. The model for Noorden's insistence on medicalized diet rests on his experience with diabetics. Defined as a disease of diet in the age before Frederick Grant Banting and Charles Herbert Best discovered insulin in 1921, diabetes seemed only to be controlled (if at all) through diet. As early as the work of John Rollo in 1796 it was clear that the reduction of carbohydrates in the diet would reduce the amount of sugar in the urine. As a result, Rollo urged that diabetics consume only meat and fat. In 1865, Apollinaire Bouchardat in Paris suggested that all foodstuffs should be reduced, including fats. As a result of the latter view, Edgar Allen created a radical hunger cure for the control of diabetes, which also functioned as a radical cure for overweight. Noorden supported the "Allen Cure," but in 1902 he made his own breakthrough in the dieting culture when he discovered that oatmeal (paired with a bit of butter and some plant protein) would reduce sugar levels. Ironically, it duplicated a fad diet of the time.

Noorden's understanding of diabetes rested on his grasp of the metabolic underpinnings of the disease, which became more and more evident during his academic life. Yet one must not forget that diabetes also came to be considered the disease of modern life. Only through diet could the disease be controlled, and weight came to be a symbol of that which had to be conquered. From the nineteenth century, diabetes had been seen as a disease of the obese and, in an odd set of associations, the Jew was implicated as obese due to an apparent increased presence of diabetes among Jews in Central Europe. (At that time no distinction had yet been made between "juvenile" and "adult-onset" diabetes.) According to Noorden, mainly rich Jewish men were fat.[9] The Jews of Western Europe were seen as those who suffered most from the pressures and speed of "modern life." Rather than arguing for any inborn metabolic inheritance of a predisposition to diabetes, Noorden stated that it was the fault of poor diet among the rich—too much rich food and alcohol, this being yet another stereotype of the Jew. This view argued against an inherited predisposition of the Jews for specific illness because of their racial inheritance, for racial thought was also an inherent part of the new biology of the late nineteenth century. The British eugenicist George Pitt-Rivers attributed the increased rate of diabetes among the Jews to "the passionate nature of their temperaments." He noted that by the 1920s diabetes was commonly called a "Jewish disease."[10] For him the Jews were inherently diseased, a quality that distinguished them from the "healthy" peoples of Europe and defined them as part of an inferior racial group. Race, in the broadest sense, became one of the explanations for what caused obesity. Not inheritance but lifestyle meant that the Jews were obese as well as diabetic: "All observers are agreed that Jews are specially liable to become diabetic...A person belonging to the richer classes in towns usually eats too much, spends a great part of his life indoors; takes too little bodily exercise, and overtaxes his nervous system in the pursuit of knowledge, business, or pleasure... Such a description is a perfectly accurate account of the well-to-do Jew, who raises himself easily by his superior mental ability to a comfortable social position, and notoriously avoids all kinds of bodily exercise."[11] It is also a comment on character.

New treatments were introduced to deal with the question of obesity, no matter what its origin. And one of the means that quickly found advocates did not depend on the compliance of the patient (as did diet and exercise). In 1909, the radiologist Jean-Alban Bergonié (1857–1925) advocated the employment of electricity to create a general sense of stimulation of the body to improve overall health. Electrification of the muscles was understood to be a surrogate for exercise. The treatment for obesity was the rapid contraction of the muscles of the body to maximize muscle strengthening while minimizing "one cannot say pain, for there is no pain with this treatment—sensation."[12]

In this treatment the patient is seated in a "semi-reclining chair" with fixed electrodes and is outfitted with a set of moveable, very large electrodes on the thigh, calf, abdomen, and arms. All are covered with damp towels to enhance conduction. The patient is covered with sacks of sand weighing up to 200 lb. Treatments last from forty minutes to sixty minutes. According to the advocates of this approach, patients lose weight and gain "general well-being." In one case cited, a patient lost 1.5 inches around his neck, as well as 3 inches from his waist in three weeks. The fact that he only lost 7 lb. suggested that he had gained muscle mass. While it was recommended that fruit, vegetables, and salad be consumed, diet was seen as a minor aspect of the overall treatment. In addition, electrotherapy is often used to treat what is seen as the pathological results of obesity, the "failure or perversion of nutrition," including diabetes.[13] Such therapies were understood as modern and

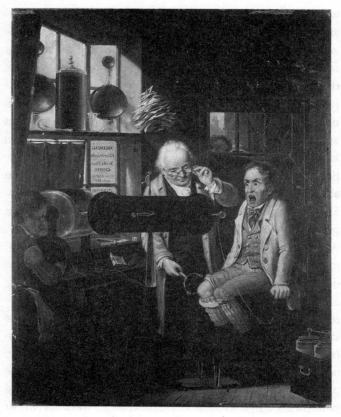

12. Edmund Bristow, "Dispensing of Medical Electricity." Oil painting (1824). (*Wellcome Collection*)

cutting edge. John Harvey Kellogg, the advocate of new, modern, machine-made health food, installed electrotherapeutic couches in his Battle Creek Sanitarium.

There was a powerful edge to the claims of electrotherapy. If obesity was primarily a process that could be reversed by a form of passive exercise then its harmful side effects could be ameliorated. Many physicians of the time came to doubt the very premise of electrotherapy. The neurologist (and later creator of psychoanalysis) Sigmund Freud (1856–1939) recalled that he "felt absolutely helpless after the disappointing results [of electrotherapy...The] successes of electrical treatment in nervous patients are the results of suggestion [...]"[4] Freud was among a growing number of physicians in the 1890s who found electrotherapy unsuccessful, yet its powerful associations with the newest technologies of mass electrification allowed electrotherapy to remain seductive until World War II. The electrotherapy of obesity seems to have had a similar placebo effect to that suspected by Freud in his patients. According to electrotherapists, patients were concerned with improvement in their general appearance and saw the physical discomfort as vital to the perceived gain.

Other aspects of the newest technologies of the late nineteenth century were, however, just as quickly adapted to the study of body weight and health. William Bradford Cannon (1871–1945) graduated from Harvard College in 1896, where he had studied with the psychologist William James and the physiologist Charles B. Davenport (with whom he had published a paper as an undergraduate). He took his MD at Harvard and worked there from 1896 in the laboratory of Henry Pickering Bowditch (1840–1911). Bowditch had recently introduced modern physiological research, developed by the German physiologist and psychologist Wilhelm Wundt, into the United States. In 1902, Cannon became an assistant professor of physiology, and in 1906 he succeeded Bowditch as the George Higginson Professor of Physiology, a position he would hold until 1942.

Under Bowditch Cannon began to investigate swallowing and stomach motility using the newly discovered X-ray techniques. Wilhelm Röntgen had discovered X-rays on December 9, 1896; not a year later Cannon was using them to trace the passage of a pearl button through the digestive system of a dog. Moving to human subjects, he found that he was able to correlate feelings of satiety with physiological responses. In 1911 he co-authored a study with Arthur Lawrence Washburn, which showed that stomach contractions were linked with hunger. Every morning Washburn, then a medical student, swallowed a length of rubber tubing, to which was tied a condom, and recorded when he felt hungry, while he went about his usual activities. The condom was filled with air, and the tubing attached to a pressure gage. The pressure gage recorded Washburn's stomach contractions and Cannon found that Washburn's hunger pangs were correlated with his sense of hunger. This study would be the most influential study about appetite for fifty years. It was later discovered that there was no causal relationship between these two feelings, as they were both caused by a drop in blood glucose levels. Cannon also published one of the earliest dieting articles in the very first issue of the *American Journal of Physiology* in 1898, recounting his research on swallowing and stomach motility.

Cannon's published books include *Bodily Changes in Pain, Hunger, Fear, and Rage* (1915) and *The Wisdom of the Body* (1932). During World War I he published widely on shock among soldiers and documented the ways in which the body's systems changed in response to shock. He argued strongly for Claude Bernard's theory of homeostasis, which explained the self-correction of bodily systems, now applied to hunger and digestion.

Thus the science of nutrition arises in the nineteenth century in the wake of discoveries concerning body chemistry of all forms, from the endocrine system to vitamin deficiency diseases. Lulu Hunt Peters MD (1873–1930), an American physician, was credited with first suggesting calorie counting as a means of gaining and losing weight. Peters served as chairman of the Public Health Committee of the California Federation of Women's Clubs in Los Angeles. She is the author of the first bestselling American diet book, *Dieting and Health, With Key to the Calories*, published in 1918. Framed as a response to World War I (and dedicated to Herbert Hoover, whose claim to fame at that point was that he "fed starving Belgium") it set out obesity as a "crime to hoard food" for which one would be fined or imprisoned. "How dare you hoard food when our nation needs it?"[15] The book is said to have sold two million copies and was published in more than 55 editions by 1939. As the model for recent modern diet books, it was directed and marketed primarily at women, written in a popular style, and included testimonials of successful weight loss.

Peters is the first major woman's voice, at a point after the beginning of the twentieth century where obesity ceased being a "man's" disease and became a disease of "women." While obese women had always been the concern of medicine, as obesity was seen as an impediment to child bearing (from the ancient Greeks to the nineteenth century), after the beginning of a systematic movement for the social and political emancipation of women in the course of the latter nineteenth century and the creation of the "New Woman," now more and more claiming control over her own body, obesity came to be defined primarily as a problem of women and thus became associated more and more with cultural notions of "vanity." Thus, unlike modern diet books, Peters included suggestions for weight control as well as beauty tips, such as how to eliminate wrinkles. Bodily control meant defining the overweight (and severely underweight) woman's body as the exemplary case of lack of will.

Dr. Peters was "overweight" herself, apparently 220 lb. (15 stones 10 lb.) at her heaviest, and claimed to have lost 70 lb. (5 stones) following her own plan. She writes, "All my life [I fought] the too, too solid. Why, I can remember when I was a child I was always being consoled by being told that I would outgrow it, and that when I matured I would have some shape...I was a delicate slip of one hundred sixty-five when I was taken [in marriage]."[16] Her "key to the calories" was an extensive list of food portions adding up to 100 calories. On a 1,200 calorie per day diet, a dieter could have twelve 100-calorie units of food. Much of her book consisted of lists of foods and their caloric content. Her system was premised on the idea of an ideal weight, for which she provided tools of measurement. The formula consisted of taking the number of inches over five feet of one's height, multiplying that number by 5.5 and adding 110. The equation was meant to yield the ideal weight, in pounds, of a "normal" woman. The number of calories a dieter was meant to consume depended upon how far their actual weight exceeded the ideal for their height. Peters dismissed the notion that fat people (women) were overindulgent or lazy; rather she divided the world into those whose metabolism quickly or slowly burned fat. She argued that even eating a bird seed if your metabolism was slow would add fat to your body. She admitted that there were those with pathologies, such as those of the thyroid, who became fat and could be cured by curing their illness, but most fat people became fat from "overeating and underexercising."[17]. This de-stigmatizing position stressed the difference of obese bodies from those of individuals who were "naturally thin."

Sir Frederick Gowland Hopkins, (1861–1947), who won the Nobel Prize for Medicine and Physiology in 1929 for his work in nutrition, saw this new science as setting the stage for all those interested in bodily systems. In his 1932 Gluckstein Lecture on "Chemistry and Life" he presented a scientific approach to the biochemistry of "living systems [that] should sometimes occupy the thought of every chemist."[18] This view, based on Hopkins' understanding of the complexity of nature, placed the living organism again into the realm of biochemistry, which had, by the 1930s, begun to see itself as concerned with the molecular level and as a science separate from any explanation of how actual systems work in living organisms. This return to a world originating in the biochemistry laboratories of Justus von Liebig (1803–73) meant a focus on processes such as metabolism in plants and animals.[19] Liebig had begun with an understanding of how such processes were carried out and Hopkins wished to return to this earlier model. Nutrition, the "intensive studies of plant and animal products," meant a return to the science that created the modern concern with diet. We now "know that the consumption of so much protein, fat, and carbohydrate lead to the excretion of so much urea and so much carbon dioxide..." But this tells us "nothing of that succession of complex events intervening between consumption and excretion, which it is the business of the biochemist to understand." This, he points out in 1932, is the goal of biochemistry as it examines the "intact and living body."[20]

Yet the idea, so potent in the explanation of the successes and failure of electrotherapy, that it was not the body that demanded treatment but rather the mind or the psyche also had older roots. As we have seen, obesity was long thought to exemplify a "failure of the will," to use the common nineteenth-century term. The will enables the rational mind to control the body. By the nineteenth century the view that it is the will that needed to be healed became the cause for that disease that is seen as the antithesis of obesity, Sir William Gull's (1816–1890) *anorexia nervosa*—the term he coined in 1874. This was a disease of the mind (rather than the will), which was "emaciation as a result of severe emotional disturbance" and "a perversion of the ego."[21] Obesity also came to be understood in precisely these terms when it fell under the treatment of the psychia-trists of the day who employed the cutting-edge somatic therapies of the day, including electrotherapy, to treat illness of the will. For the will or the psyche came more and more to be understood as a product of the body, as in Carl Vogt's (1817–1895) mid-century turn of phrase, that mind is to brain as bile is to liver.

There was a powerful alternative to such somatizing views in the arguments that were presented in the 1930s within psychoanalysis, then at the peak of its influence in the United States. The prime figure in arguing for a psychogenic model for obesity was Hilde Bruch (1904–84) who escaped the Nazis to England and then to Lulu Peter's America and ended her career as Professor of Psychiatry at Baylor Medical School. She popularized Gull's diagnosis of anorexia nervosa and was a frequently cited specialist on obesity who revolu-tionized the debate between those who saw exogenous or endogenous causes for obesity. She provided the first complex psychological theory of obesity—seeing obesity as arising in the child through pathologies in the family rather

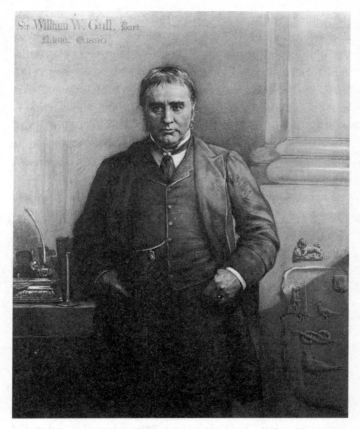

13. Sir William Withey Gull. Photogravure by Duclaud after Elliot & Fry. (*Wellcome Collection*)

than as a somatic problem in the individual. The debate of the Enlightenment, whether it is nature or nurture that makes the obese, by the mid-twentieth century comes to be a debate between the pathologies of the body and those of the psyche.

Bruch's claim to fame is that she popularized the diagnosis of anorexia nervosa. Yet she was, during her lifetime, an often-cited specialist on obesity who provided the first complex psychological theory of obesity—linking its appearance to the world of the pathological family. Her interest in obesity seems to have begun with her arrival in the United States in 1934, where according to her own account she was amazed at the huge number of fat, truly corpulent children, not only in the clinics but also on the street, in the subway, and in the schools.[22] Her work on the "psychosomatic aspects of obesity" was funded by the Josiah Macy, Jr. Foundation and the results from this began to appear in the 1940s and were summarized by her in her book of 1973, *Eating Disorders,* where obesity is defined as a state that develops through specific family interaction beginning at birth. The core of the book is her view of the child's struggle to develop autonomy in the family setting, a view championed by Theodore Lidz (who created the theory of the "schizophrenogenic mother") with whom she had worked in Baltimore between 1941 and 1943. Undergoing a training analysis with Frieda Fromm-Reichmann in Washington at the time, she began to see more complex readings of the work on obesity than those that had brought her to Fromm-Reichmann's initial attention.

Typical of Bruch's readings of obesity is the case study of a 4½-year-old girl weighing 90 lb (6 stones 6 lb.). The child had been accidentally conceived during the war and was initially rejected by her mother.[23] For the mother, "feeding showed love and expiation of guilt"[24] for rejecting the very idea of bearing the child. The mother is a compulsive confabulator, always embellishing the tales she tells about her daughter's treatments in order to manipulate her daughter's treatment. Bruch thus provides obese children with a childhood of rejection that explains their obesity. Now Bruch's child is female, following World War I, the exemplary patient in questions of obesity shifts from the male (where it had been since the ancient Greeks) to the female with the construction of the image of the "New Woman." But this has a special role in Bruch's system. Here it is the mother who is the cause of the child's obesity. The child's obesity is a neurotic response to her mother's "unnatural" rejection of her.

Yet little is known of Bruch's initial work on obesity. In her 1928 dissertation, written under the renowned pediatrician Carl Noeggerath at Freiburg im Breisgau, she tested the stamina and lung capacity of children with the newly developed spirometer. She traced how their respiration increased with increased work (turning a weighted wheel). One of the children, Maria O., was, according to Bruch, chronically obese, weighing 58.4 kg (127 lb 4 oz.) at the age of 12. She "speaks tiredly and in a monotone, complains about constant tiredness and weakness of memory. There is neither determination nor a joy for work."[25] This case study provides all of the negative images about desire and work and intelligence that are found in classic images of obese children. But it is also the classic racist image of the non-productive "fat" Jew that haunts the medical texts of her time, where the "Jew" remained the prime example of obesity.

Bruch also provides a rationale of the psychological state of the obese child; the absence of the love of the mother, the negation of the natural desire of the parent for the offspring. The image of the lazy, stupid fat child comes now with a family that can neither love nor desire. Bruch offers an alternative model for exogenous obesity—one beyond the control of the individual and, more importantly, beyond racial categories. Any child raised badly can (indeed will) become obese.

Bruch had been raised in a religious German-Jewish household and attended a one-room Jewish elementary school in the tiny mainly Catholic hamlet of Dülkens in 1910. She was of the very first generation of young women who forced their way into the academic *Gymnasium* (for her in Gladbach)—rather than the traditional *Höhere Mädchenschule*. She had wanted to become a mathematician but settled for the more pragmatic study of medicine. In 1923, she entered the world of somatic medicine in Würzburg and then, in 1924, studied in Freiburg, where she wrote her thesis. This world demanded an understanding of the inherent relationship between race and obesity. All of the discussions about Jews and diabetes, obesity, and food were part of the medical discourse about eating disorders that shaped her professional training. It was this world that Bruch rebelled against, especially after fleeing Nazi Germany, where the notion of race and hygiene was so explicitly stated within the medical world. Bruch's construction of an alternative, psychological, model ran against the dominant racial model in Germany but also the implications of the metabolic model that held sway in the United States when she arrived. Psychoanalysis provided a non-racial, non-biological answer to what had been a racial or biological explanation.

Sigmund Freud had shown that "race," a staple of the cutting edge medical science of Vienna in his day, was not a factor in either somatic or psychological illnesses of his day. As early as the 1890s Freud had argued for a universal model to explain that "the relation between body and mind (in animals no less than in human beings)" is as much

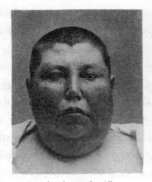
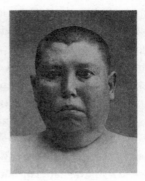

Avant le traitement thyroïdien.
Poids : 156 kilos.

Après le traitement thyroïdien.
Poids : 123 kilos.

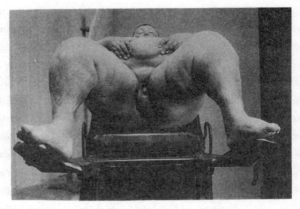

INFANTILISME (TYPE BRISSAUD) ET DÉGÉNÉRESCENCE PSYCHIQUE
(*Magalhaes Lemos.*)

Facies lunaire. Arrêt de développement des organes génitaux. Absence des caractères
sexuels secondaires.

14. A man, aged 37, suffering from 'infantilism' (Type Brissaud) and a physical degenerative disorder—possibly thyroid. First image taken before thyroid treatment, second, after, and the third of the man lying in an obsterics/ gynecologist's chair with legs apart revealing lack of secondary sexual characteristics in genital area. From: *Nouvelle Iconographie de la Salpêtrieré; Clinique des Maladies du Système Nerveux* (Paris: LeCrosnier et Babe, Libraires-Editeurs, Place de L'Ecole de Medecine, 1906). (*Wellcome Collection*)

determined by "mind" as it is by "body," that it "is a reciprocal one." Patients whose illnesses are psychogenic have constantly shifting symptoms, which included responses to food: "A patient who has hitherto been incapacitated by headaches but has had a fairly good digestion may next day enjoy a clear head but may thenceforward be unable to manage most kinds of food. Again, his sufferings may suddenly cease if there is a marked change in the circumstances of his existence. If he is travelling he may feel perfectly well and be able to enjoy the most varied diet without any ill effects, but when he gets home he may once more have to restrict himself to sour milk."[26] Freud is not interested in questions of body size here but the notion that all symptoms, including eating disorders, have the possibility of being transformed into new but relevant symptoms: a notion that is central to his theory of psychopathology.

Bruch's work trumped earlier psychoanalytic approaches to obesity, such as that of the Viennese psychoanalyst and psychosomaticist Felix Deutsch (1884–1964), which were anchored in Freud's views concerning the relative stability of symptoms. He stressed the interchangeability of overweight with other somatic symptoms. Very much in the model of traditional psychoanalysis, obesity was but one symptom of an underlying neurosis that could easily be transformed into other pathological mental states:

> Suppose that a female patient comes to consult us believing herself to be suffering from obesity and demands treatment to reduce her weight. It would be incumbent upon us, not only to prescribe a suitable diet, but to recognize that while by dietetic methods we can certainly influence the body, the prohibition of certain foods cannot fail to reactivate all

the unconscious fantasies connected with the oral zone. We know, for instance, that certain states of depression (ranging in degree up to the severest forms) manifest themselves in the form of disturbances in the taking of food, and that these disturbances are connected with the introjection of the lost love object and with severe feelings of culpability, which derive from the attitude to the introjected object. If we were to treat such a patient by the inconsiderate prohibition of certain articles of diet, we might very well find that she would be led to react with an onset of severe depressive states. Not only are there certain patients who tell us that they always become extremely "nervous" when they try to diet strictly, we actually encounter some in whom an attack of depression has ensued immediately after the enforcement of a reducing diet. Thus now a day's medical treatment is being influenced by considerations of an entirely new order.[27]

Indeed, the Viennese psychoanalyst Franz Wittels (1880–1950), one of Freud's original followers, was convinced that even "beauty" could be one of those symptoms that paralleled obesity: "I became acquainted with a family in which a number of children had to undergo treatment because of neurotic disturbances. A brother suffered from obsessional ideas, another was a schizophrenic, a third showed pathological obesity, and one of the sisters at the age of puberty 'burst out' into glorious beauty, flamboyant with sex appeal, large sensual eyes, vivid colouring, tall slender body."[28] Obesity was not a primary sign of any specific psychopathological problem and could not be treated as such. It was clearly not to be treated by somatic interventions, such as dieting, because it was not only a psychogenetic response but could easily be transformed into other symptoms. Wittels' family of neurotics presented obesity and narcissistic beauty as equal psychopathological states.

All of this changed with Hilde Bruch's championing of a family-based definition of obesity that dominated the discussion in the United States after the 1940s. Obesity came to stand for a specific error in "mothering," which reflected the developmental problems of the specific individual. Eating disorders (for later Bruch's interests expanded into the field of anorexia) exhibit the primary symptoms resulting from a specific set of the psychological state of the parent not of the child. All of her patients suffered from some developmental disruption in infancy, as the child focused on oral gratification and the bonding with the mother. Inappropriate feeding or rejection by the mother in this early stage led to a pathological relationship with food. Such symptoms could not easily be transformed into other, analogous somatic problems. As A. H. Vander, in 1944, summarizing Bruch's views, for the broader psychoanalytic community noted:

> The dominant emotional patterns in the children consisted of aggressive demands on the mother for feeding, dressing, and toilet care; avoidance of physical activity, sports, and social contacts; greed in areas other than food (e.g., addiction to movies); and lack of open aggression to persons other than the mother. None of the children ate a well-balanced diet and generally they preferred starches. The family patterns were quite uniform. In general, the fathers were weak and unaggressive. The mothers frequently gave histories of early emotional deprivation, poverty, and hunger. Their attitudes toward the children were ambivalent, combining overprotection and anxiety with overt hostility at the child's demands. The mothers consciously hoped to possess the exclusive love of their children by keeping them in a state of perpetual babyhood. They actively encouraged the children to overeat. Food

seemed to symbolize love to both mother and child and also acted as a reassurance to the child against many anxieties arising from his social ostracism and his sexual conflicts. The author believes that such children enjoy their obesity and utilize it to fantasize that they are big, powerful, and therefore safe. She concludes that, "Obesity in childhood represents a disturbance in personality in which excessive bodily size becomes the expressive organ of the conflict." Dr. Bruch is to be highly commended for placing the study of obesity on a rational basis.[29]

Psychoanalytic work on obesity thereafter rested on Bruch's "rational" model of neurosis and its family connection. This model reflects as much the obese children's choice of foods as their psychological attitude toward their bodies. Fat people were made as children. Fat was a sign of early psychological distress not physiological pathologies, whether systemic or inherited. Such patients, as one paper of 1970 noted, "become obese partly in relation to over-nutrient influences in foetal life or early childhood. Such influences will sometimes have had neurotic determinants based in the mother, in the family, and in the specific maternal attitude to the patient as an infant."[30] The fact is that they can undo this influence: "Some patients, despite remaining massively obese for the meantime, may have the capacity to make a more healthy social adjustment auguring better for the future. The male patient and our last case seem to demonstrate this." The obese patient can be saved in terms of these psychodynamic models of obesity. The baneful influence of the mother can be undone. No such possibility exists for the racial model of obesity. For the racial predisposition to obesity will out, no matter what level of self-control is exerted.

Such psychoanalytic explanations continued to fascinate. Bruch's view dominated the accounts of obesity in the 1940s.[31] Even though C. M. Louttit, in his classic *Clinical Psychology of Children's Behavior Problems* in 1947, stated that, "Of course, many if not most obese children are suffering from endocrinopathies and are not primarily nutritional disorders."[32] The psychological causation was dominant, as an anonymous reviewer of Louttit noted that year: "This was disproven by Bruch and others prior to World War II and the importance of psychological mechanisms in the production of obesity in children has been amply demonstrated."[33] Psychodynamic explanations dominated, as Gustav Bychowski argued in his account of a neurotic obesity that he viewed as "an autoplastic materialization, unconscious impulses using the body rather than external reality as a medium for expression and alteration."[34] For women, he sees such an obsessive impulse as linked to "early fixations on the preambivalent oral level, identification with both parental love objects, regression, and reactivation of oral drives aiming at partial incorporation with resulting denial of true femininity, and trends toward masculinization." The difficulty of seeing this as a problem inherent in female sexuality haunted mainstream psychoanalysis at a time when obesity came to be understood in the medical as well as the broader culture as a "woman's problem."

Yet this approach never quite vanished from within psychoanalytic discourse, even though some work in the 1970s postulated a post-oral phase origin in the Oedipal conflict, sibling rivalry, or even early childhood sexuality. In 1971, a study reported on a case in which pregnancy and lactation was accompanied by an awareness of a childhood fascination with reproduction as an explanation for obesity:

As the regression deepened, her Oedipal fantasies faded into the background and she engaged in much projection and introjection. She was continually preoccupied with her lactating breasts, which were a source of pride and pleasure to her. Daily she expressed the milk, noting its color, consistency, and taste…She also thought that in order to grow big and have a baby inside her, she must eat a great deal and not allow feces or urine to escape (a conjecture that had contributed to her moderate obesity); any act of elimination was accompanied by intense anxiety and with-holding.[35]

The focus on the infantile is reflected in further case studies in the age of AIDS, where perhaps a more subtle understanding of ethnicity and its reading in American culture could have been undertaken.

An obese, handsome 5-year-old, José was brought to the clinic by his foster mother because of his aggressive, self-destructive outbursts. The most severe of these culminated in José's puncturing his arm with pins. José's mother had been imprisoned for selling drugs, and the boy's care had been entrusted to his father and paternal grandmother. He was routinely beaten for infractions of the house rules, and his daily needs, such as food and clothing, were not always fulfilled. His father, who reportedly was himself obese and unkempt, contracted AIDS through intravenous (IV) drug use. When word got out that his father was ill with AIDS, José was teased by his peers and quietly ostracized by the staff…José's profound feelings of abandonment and victimization seemed to result in his defensive identification with the powerful, deserting (through illness and death) parent—the aggressor. José's obesity also appeared to be in part a way of maintaining a tie to his dead father, perhaps due to a primitive identification, a result of fusion of self and object images.[36]

It is clear that the interfamilial structures still determine obesity in this model; not any ethnic or "racial" quality.

Bruch's views shaped the medical discourse on obesity as much as did her work on anorexia nervosa. Indeed, as late as 1992, her work on obesity as a product of psychodynamic forces is used to provide an explanation for the presence of precisely the opposite: eating disorders, such as anorexia nervosa.[37] But of equal importance was the fact that she wrote widely for popular "woman's magazines" and served as the advisor of weight questions to the most popular newspaper "agony aunt" Ann Landers. Bruch's views, shaped against the world of a moral panic about Jewish difference, came to create a model for obesity rooted in the individual experience of the patient in the context of the family—not a race. Bruch's world view permitted a new, if also troubling, redefinition of obesity in its relationship to mental states. But it also allowed for the possibility of "cure" or at least treatment through psychological rather than physiological intervention. We have not come very far from this view in our public outcry about the epidemic of obesity today. We seek a new type of magic bullet to ward off the collapse of the nation. Obesity remains a "moral panic" as the obese represent as true a threat to the national states as Bruch's concern with the family pointed to the focus in the 1960s and 1970s with the "death of the family." Such a view had a real impact in the shift within the African-American community in understanding excessive body size not as beautiful or healthy but as a disease process that originated within the family and led to multiple somatic illnesses. The public discussion of the collapse of the "black family" was the major precursor for the shift within that community toward seeing body size as a marker of illness.[38] In the United States, it was the "death of the nuclear family" that was seen as the potential cause of massive social unrest within African-American society as the often quoted work of the sociologist Daniel Patrick Moynihan stressed in 1965: "From the wild Irish slums of the nineteenth-century Eastern seaboard, to the riot-torn suburbs of Los Angeles, there is one unmistakable lesson in American history; a community that allows a large number of men to grow up in broken families, dominated by women, never acquiring any stable relationship to male authority, never acquiring any set of rational expectations about the future—that community asks for and gets chaos. Crime, violence, unrest, disorder—most particularly the furious, unrestrained lashing out at the whole social structure—that is not only to be expected; it is very near to inevitable. And it is richly deserved."[39] But it was the social meaning attached to the "collapsing" black family that was seen as the cause of social change, just as the collapse of the family order explained obesity and other eating disorders for Hilde Bruch.

With the decline of the power of psychogenetic explanations for mental illnesses in the late twentieth century, deeply psychological explanations of obesity tended to vanish. Contemporary psychiatry does not consider "simple obesity" as "consistently associated with a psychological or behavioral syndrome."[40] Today, psychiatry speaks of obsessive-compulsive disorders or addiction to food.[41] In most cases it places the desire to eat beyond the control of the individual. In such cases, behavioral therapy, such as a twelve-step program (Food Addicts Anonymous) is proposed, analogous to the control (rather than the treatment) of alcoholism (through Alcoholics Anonymous).

But by 2008 the blame game had moved substantially from bad parenting to bad genes. A British study published in 2008

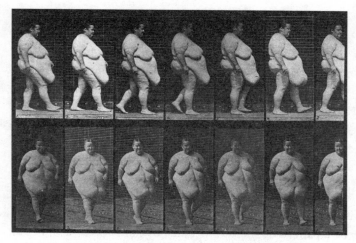

15. Eadweard Muybridge, "A Gargantuan Woman Walking." Collotype (1887) (Philadelphia: The Photo-Gravure Company: 1887). (*Wellcome Collection*)

in the *American Journal of Clinical Nutrition* found that differences in body mass index and waist size were 77% governed by genes.[42] Even good parenting cannot answer that claim. For all of these views, "fat" still points toward social as well as personal catastrophe with a single cause that could be identified and treated. Neither parenting nor genetics seem truly to play much of a role in our debate about personal responsibility versus external causation. All such approaches to obesity see it as a symptom of a single, underlying pathological problem.

In the late twentieth century certain forms of psychotherapy, such as behavioral therapy, have been more recently employed to facilitate weight loss. Indeed, "body image treatment" through "cognitive behavioral therapy" has become a commonplace in the self-treatment of both over- and underweight since the development in the mid-1980s of Jonathan Butters and

Thomas Cash's approach.[43] Cash's audiotape program *Body-Image Therapy: A Program for Self-Directed Change*, while aimed at mental health practitioners, set the stage for self-treatment by those women who desired to change their own negative body image. Other non-clinical settings, such as weight loss support groups, also use a psychotherapeutic model to enable the loss of weight. Experts suggest that behavioral therapy is a good non-surgical alternative when it comes to weight loss; the results, however, are not always long-lived. While there is an average weight reduction of 7–10% of initial body weight during the first twenty-four weeks of treatment, further treatment seems to offer little further weight loss. Indeed there seems to be a pattern of relapse attributed by behavioral therapists to their patient's "inability to maintain the strategies they learned in treatment." Given that such strategies are to change behavioral patterns, it seems that long-term efficacy is unlikely.

Behavioral techniques rest on the claim that obese people gain weight either as a response to conditioned learning or environmental stimuli or as a coping mechanism in response to stress and arousal. Thus therapy can include stimulus control (controlling the presence of certain "trigger" foods in the home, and increasing the presence of exercise cues), problem-solving strategies, social assertion (figuring out ways to assert one's dietary philosophy in an uncongenial environment), setting short-term goals to enhance positive thinking, cognitive reconditioning to help alter negative thought patterns, relapse prevention (learning to gage which situations are detrimental to weight loss commitments) and building a support network.

Therapy for eating disorders has now reached into the world of the Internet. There is the claim that Internet-driven intervention combined with individual therapy is more effective than therapy alone. Such on-line activities tend, it is claimed, to reduce clients' anxiety about how they appear and are being judged, since they are unseen by the therapist. The use of on-line behavioral therapy together with on-line virtual reality has been claimed to modify the body awareness and thus impact on problematic social and eating behaviors.[44]

A comparative study, which assigned some volunteers to Weight Watchers and others to a self-help group for weight loss, found that clients who attended Weight Watchers had a greater tendency to lose weight.[45] The researchers concluded that this was because of the behavioral component of the program, which was actively reinforced through group meetings and weekly weigh-ins. Dieting, they found, could only have long-term results if it was part of a larger lifestyle philosophy, instead of a compartmentalized activity one undertook merely to lose weight. Another study, conducted by scientists at Baylor, analysed the difference between two types of treatment for women engaged in binge eating: one involved dieting and behavioral therapy, while the other consisted only of behavioral therapy measures.[46] What the research team found six months after the treatment program was that the women who dieted and had therapy had lost about 0.6 kg, while those who only had therapy had gained about 1.3 kg. What these women had experienced was a marked reduction in their binge-eating patterns. An eighteen-month follow-up examination revealed that both groups had once again gained weight, but that there had been an overall reduction in binge eating. The researchers once again concluded the ineffectuality of dieting as a weight loss measure, but saw that other behavioral patterns, such as binge eating, had undergone a significant change.

When weight gain or loss is considered to be a psychological illness rather than a behavioral aberration, very different approaches are used. Certainly, the use of "talk-therapy," whether in the form of classic psychoanalysis or short-term psychotherapy has a long history. Indeed, family therapy remains a mainstay for the treatment of eating disorders, such as bulimia and anorexia nervosa, but it is used relatively rarely as a treatment for obesity. Alternative psychoanalytic explanations, such as libido theory, have been offered to explain the presence of obesity. The effectiveness of interpersonal psychotherapy has been claimed by Christopher Fairburn as an answer to the lack of long-term effectiveness of behavioral therapy.[47] One large-scale study in 1977 tracked the treatment of 84 obese patients (paired with 63 normal-weight patients) treated with a wide range of psychoanalytic approaches. The resultant (short-term) weight loss was seen to be approximately the same as for those patients treated specifically for weight loss.[48]

With the reappearance of "Body Dysmorphic Disorder" as a major diagnosis for certain forms of mental illness in the standard American handbook of mental illnesses (the *DSM-IV-TR*) and the championing of this by American psychiatry, the relationship between eating disorders (also a psychiatric category) and body dysmorphic disorder has been raised. "Dysmorphophobia" is a diagnostic category coined by the Italian psychiatrist Enrico Morselli (1852–1929) in 1891. Given that the treatment of choice of the latter is the prescription of serotonin-reuptake inhibitors, a class of psychotropic drugs, one can imagine the use of such interventions in the treatment of eating disorders. Thus, weight loss (and gain) comes to be understood as a somatic rather than a psychological disorder.

Even in the application of alternative approaches to weight loss, such as mental imagery, there is a neurological claim for efficacy. Imaging is "'seeing' in the absence of actual visual sensory inputs" and is claimed to activate the dopamine-reward pathway and thus enhance weight loss.[49] The creation of "aversive imagery," such as "disgusting images" of "rat droppings in chocolate chip cookies" seems to be effective in weight reduction.[50] Such approaches have a wide range of therapeutic modalities. As early as 1843, hypnotism was used to "control a female patient's appetite for certain foods which exacerbated dyspepsia in her."[51] By the 1960s, hypnotism (now restored to clinical acceptability) reappeared for the treatment of overweight.

The battle between those who see obesity as a mental health issue with somatic symptoms and those who see it as a somatic illness with psychological symptoms is ongoing. Depending on the specialist's view, obesity is treated in radically different ways. This could be seen as a sign that obesity is a truly multi-factorial disease process, or that it is a symptom of quite different and mutually exclusive causes.

VI

NEW CAUSES; NEW SOLUTIONS FOR OBESITY

With the rise of women's emancipation in the West (as well as in China and Japan) in the course of the nineteenth century, the standard model for the study of the relationship between sex and obesity focused on women's bodies. While in the 1940s Jean Vague had introduced the differentiation between "android" and "gynoid" obesity, men were only an afterthought.[1] For Vague, men were apple-shaped (they carried their fat abdominally) and women were pear-shaped (they carried their fat in the buttocks, hips, and thighs). But it was not the physiological difference between the sexes that dominated the popular as well as the medical discourses on obesity. The women's movement of the post-World-War-II generation came to see fat not as a physiological but as a social-psychological phenomenon in the light of psychogenetic models otherwise being abandoned within the allopathic medicine of the day. The central theme of much of this work has focused on how patriarchal society (men) abhors fat women and thus causes all women to hate their own bodies. In this rhetoric, no woman's body could be slim enough. Fat, as Susie Orbach wrote thirty years ago, is a feminist issue.[2]

Kim Chernin coined the phrase a "tyranny of slenderness" to reflect Western society's growing preoccupation with thinness and the attendant issues for the fat female body.[3] While this social and psychological cause remains a focus of popular concern, a wide range of new explanations and causes for obesity arose in response. Social pressures (as with the arguments about obesity in the African-American community) were at fault for a distorted body image. While this view continued within popular culture, the abandonment of somatic explanations for obesity gave rise to a new science of obesity that draws on cutting edge developments in human biology, whether or not these developments were completely appropriate for an understanding of weight.

What has obesity become in the twenty-first century? Certainly it is no longer the disease of patriarchy. It seems to have a simple definition today as a "complex disorder with a deceptively simple ultimate cause: the prolonged consumption of calories in excess of those expended."[4] By the twenty-first century, the new global medicine of obesity stresses that there may well be a plurality of often conflicting causes of obesity.[5] Central among them, however, are genetic-physiological or sociological explanations:

1. A shift in "quality of life" and life expectancy. We live longer now, have less physically stressful occupations, and have easier access to more food. "The epidemic of obesity can be understood as a logical consequence of the fact that it has become progressively easier to consume more calories while expending fewer."[6]

2. We depend psychologically on food as a means of manipulating our immediate environment. This is an assumption that obesity is simply on a continuum with anorexia nervosa, which has been so defined by

psychologists. Obesity is thus a mental illness, but this category itself shifts from a psychological to a somatic one, as anorexia comes to be understood as a biologically determined mental illness on a continuum with depression.

3. Abundant access to poor food and the absence of structures to engage physical activity: the obesity of poverty argument.

4. The loss of control over our consumption of food because of our addictive behavior. Addiction is usually understood following the medical model of some type of pathological genetic predisposition in an individual or a group, rather than a "weakness of will."

5. A "normal" genetic predisposition understood in terms of evolutionary biological drive to accumulate body fat in order to preclude starvation in times of famine. This is the "*ob*-gene" (or "*thrifty*-gene") argument discovered in work on the genetics of obesity in mice. Its findings were then extrapolated to human beings.

6. A disruption of normal growth because of the changes in the endocrine system though pathological changes including aging (also understood as pathological).

7. The result of infection as, over the past twenty years, six different pathogens have been reported to cause obesity in animal models as well as humans.

What is clear is that any single explanation may be possible for any given individual, but it is the social implications of "obesity" that have now produced today's "epidemic" of obesity.

The anxiety about "epidemics" points to the danger that lies in the "moral panic" that defines those "diseases" we openly fear and those "infected" persons we openly disdain. Obesity is now the central danger confronting all aspects of all societies (as it is seen as an epidemic of poverty as well as affluence). The spread seems to be "like" a contagious disease. Yet each discussion of obesity seems to choose some model for the cause and nature of obesity that can be the point of intervention to end this plague. It may be the danger of fast food, too much sugar or fat, too little exercise, a damaged psyche or weak will, too large portions, genetic predisposition or hormonal imbalance. It is not surprising that there has been a strong argument for at least some cases of obesity being the result of an infectious agency— this fulfills all of the metaphoric power of the "moral panic" about fat and contains its locus to a limited and treatable cause. A "magic bullet" can be found in the new range of explanations, unlike most of the other suggested biological or social causes postulated for obesity.

In the later twentieth century, the struggle between the psychological and the physiological takes a new turn with the development of the field of the genetics of obesity, as pioneered by Jules Hirsch at Rockefeller University. New technology has allowed researchers to identify genes, which provide the blueprint necessary for the body to manufacture specific hormones, such as insulin or estrogen. These hormones tell the body to store or burn fat, carbohydrates, and protein. Additionally hormones maintain body temperature, regulate digestive rate, tell the body to stop or start eating, and initiate growth in children and adolescents. When a person does not have a gene that is essential for the production or activation of a hormone, a disease usually develops. For example, a person who lacks the gene to manufacture growth hormone (pituitin) will not be able to grow to normal heights. People can carry a gene without having the disease, which means that a child can inherit a disease that neither parent has.

As scientists discovered genes that seemed to trigger diseases such as cancer and diabetes, they began searching for genes that cause weight gain or loss as well. Genes in animals are very similar to those in humans, thus animals are frequently used to find new genes and to understand their function. In the 1990s Jeffrey Friedman (1954–) discovered the obesity regulator, leptin, by studying genetic mechanisms of weight regulation in "fat" mice.

Mice rather than "man" became the favored object of study for the genetics of obesity. In the early 1950s a naturally "fat" mouse had been "discovered" at the Jackson Laboratory in Bar Harbor, Maine. This mutant mouse was so huge that it was assumed that it was pregnant, until it was discovered that it was a male mouse. Friedman was further inspired by the work of Ethan Allen Sims, who had been exploring the link between obesity and diabetes using male inmates at the Vermont State Prison. Sims found that only very few inmates could easily put on weight and these found it the most difficult to lose it. (In the nineteenth century, obesity was found among the inhabitants of insane asylums and was attributed to their innate degeneracy.) Mice and man became linked in Friedman's research.

Friedman received national recognition after the isolation of the obesity gene (*ob*-gene) and its human homolog had been publicized.[7] Its central importance and credibility in this particular field of research is that any researcher wanting to study this gene in obese mice must have information about the gene itself. Knowing the exact code allows hypotheses to be set up about whether the physiological problem is a defect in the protein that the *ob*-gene makes, or whether it is the perhaps defective receptor of *ob* that is the problem. If genetics determines our excess weight, there seems to be no real cure, as genetic manipulation for other genetically transmitted illnesses has been generally unsuccessful. Clearly neither psychological nor endocrinological interventions would make a substantial difference if the cause of obesity were genetic.

In this case, as subsequent studies were able to confirm, there are in fact several ways of having an obese phenotype (i.e., a fat mouse). In some cases, the ob-gene itself is defective, and in others, the receptor gene is defective (a different gene, called db). Of course, other genes entirely can also cause obesity. This paper was the starting point for closer examination of what the gene products resulting in obesity are, and how they interact. The paper is credible, as the techniques used to determine this sequence are standard, universally accepted genetic methods for finding genes. The method began with recombination studies. This means that researchers allow mice to breed in large numbers and then look for inheritance patterns that do not necessarily follow Mendelian patterns. By comparing numbers of fat and lean offspring in relation to some other genetically related trait (molecular markers), it is possible to determine approximately where on a chromosome (and on which chromosome) a mutation is.

The particular chromosome and the gene's approximate location were already known to Friedman and his colleagues. The next step was to continue to determine where on the chromosome ob is by comparing it with other genes close to it (by making a genetic map, which becomes increasingly specific). After this, they had a (comparatively) very small region of DNA that they knew contained the gene, and by "insetting" the region of the chromosome into bacteria using recombinant techniques and growing the bacteria, they could see which products were expressed, and were, therefore, the result of the gene. Furthermore, the sequences were compared with standard DNA libraries to see if homology with other genes exists. In the case of Friedman's work, this technique worked because the product of the gene, a protein called leptin, was already known, and so they only had to compare the region of DNA and its putative gene product with the protein leptin to see whether they had the right region. These methods are entirely standard, and there is no reason to doubt the report's veracity. Thus, this paper is central because not only is it entirely within the bounds of standard genetic research, but it is also the starting point for any further work. However, its genetic credibility does not absolve its scientific weaknesses, namely that it equates obesity with bad health, and considers obesity the cause rather than the symptom of other illnesses.

Leptin is secreted in response to the amount of fat in the body of the animal. The release of leptin decreases appetite and tells the mouse to stop eating. If the gene producing leptin is missing or damaged, the mice will not stop eating and will gain significant amounts of body fat. When the animals are injected with leptin, they will stop eating and return to normal weight. The discovery of the function of leptin led researchers to predict that if leptin would be administered to obese individuals, they would lose weight. Despite unsuccessful clinical trials, drug companies began to market leptin in the form of over-the-counter dieting supplements like Leptoprin. The problem with these supplements is that leptin is minimally effective in controlling weight when injected and completely ineffective when taken orally. At the point of publication of this book, leptin has not yet been shown to be a useful treatment for weight loss but the research is still ongoing. A very few families have been identified who possess damaged copies of the *ob*-gene from both parents; their obesity was indeed treatable through the use of leptin.

Although leptin was not the answer to weight loss that scientists had hoped for, research continued to locate a gene that is responsible for fat gain. As with leptin, if a hormone could be discovered that reduces body weight, the pharmaceutical industry could potentially manufacture and distribute the hormone as a drug or supplement to aid in weight loss. Two hormones of interest are ghrelin, discovered in 1996, and obestatin, discovered in 2005. The role of ghrelin in obesity is not fully understood, yet obese individuals tend to have lower levels of this hormone than do non-obese people. Additionally, people suffering from anorexia nervosa tend to have higher ghrelin levels than people of normal weight. These two findings have led researchers to believe that ghrelin is an important hormone for controlling appetite. Obestatin decreases the appetite of mice and could possibly do the same in humans.

But Friedman's hypothesis did not rest with the explanation of where the genetic key to obesity in mice lay. He concludes with the evolutionary biological explanation that: "Heterozygous mutations at *ob* may provide a selective advantage in human populations subjected to caloric deprivation. Identification of *ob* offers an entry point into the pathways that regulate adiposity and body weight and should provide a fuller understanding of the pathogenesis of obesity."[8] At that point, the meanings associated with obesity shifted radically from psychological to genetic explanations. However, the genetic explanations were given an evolutionary meaning to explain their "function." Fat had to have purpose if it were an inherent part of the genome. It could not be a random or a secondary effect. It had "meaning" in the past when populations were at risk from starvation. Actually, a counter "just-so story" could be told about the fat members of prehistoric populations who were the favorite prey of saber-toothed tigers as they ran much slower.

Subsequent to defining the *ob*-gene, Friedman's laboratory found that injecting leptin into mice decreased their body weight because food intake was reduced and energy expenditure increased. As a result of Friedman's discovery, current research has been aimed at trying to understand the genetic basis of obesity in human beings and the role leptin plays in transmitting its weight-reducing signal.

The notion of giving meaning to fat in the evolutionary past made it "natural" rather than pathological. As Friedman later wrote:

> In their efforts to lose weight, obese individuals may be fighting a powerful set of evolutionary forces honed in an environment drastically different from that of today … Twin studies, adoption studies, and studies of familial aggregation confirm a major contribution of genes to the development of obesity. Indeed, the heritability of obesity is equivalent to that of height and exceeds that of many disorders for which a genetic basis is generally accepted. It is worth noting that height has also increased significantly in Western countries in the twentieth century; for example, the average US Civil War soldier was 5 ft. 4 in. tall. Yet, in contrast to the situation with obesity, most people readily accept the fact that genetic factors contribute to differences in stature.[9]

Strangely, this is analogous to the argument that Francis Galton (1822–1911), Charles Darwin's cousin and the creator of "eugenics," made in 1869 concerning the inheritability of physical characteristics. He wanted to prove that the British working class was stupid, small, and puny because of their inheritance following his dictum that "nature" outweighed "nurture" (a phrase that he coined). Even his contemporaries dismissed this, noting the radical difference in nutrition between the working class and Galton's ideal upper-middle-class Englishman.

The discovery of a genetic marker for obesity provided an answer to the notion that certain groups, such as the Jews were predisposed to obesity (and thus diabetes). (The distinction between type 1 ["juvenile"] and type 2 ["adult-onset"] diabetes was first made by Harold Percival Himsworth in 1936. Today both are understood to have a genetic component.) At the beginning of the twentieth century, scientists began to explore the relationship between the Jews' predisposition for "diabetes" and the assumed relationship between diabetes and obesity. One physician in 1926 noted that, "since one in twelve obese Gentiles develops diabetes, no less than one in eight obese Jews develop it. This, it is suggested, is to be explained by the fact that a fat Hebrew is always fatter than a fat Gentile, and that it is the higher grade of obesity which determines the Semitic preponderance in diabetes."[10] The assumption about fat and the "oriental" race is one that comes to haunt discussions of the meaning of fat.[11] When W. H. Sheldon developed his "somato-types" in the 1940s, he observed that Jews show an exaggeration in each of his body types. Thus fat Jews are somehow fatter than fat non-Jews.[12] More recent studies of obese Jews look at the complex behavior patterns that occur when religious demands for fasting and the psychological predisposition of the obese come in conflict.

Today, diabetes as a by-product of obesity is not generally considered a Jewish illness. Research now follows the so-called thrifty genotype hypothesis, which had been suggested in 1964. Simply stated, it has been observed that, when mice are transferred from a harsh to a benign environment, they gain weight and become hyperglycemic. The "*ob*-gene" was the genetic marker that showed the validity of this approach. Thus, when one measures first-generation groups of immigrants to the United States in the late nineteenth century or in Israel today, one finds a substantially higher rate of diabetes. The initial groups, as in the example of the Yemenites, who immigrated to Israel from a harsh environment, showed an extremely low index of diabetes when they arrived in Israel. This index, however, skyrocketed after just a short time of living in their new environment. Similar findings have been shown among Native Americans, when tribes were moved from hostile to less hostile environments. Thus diabetes and obesity seem to be the index of a failure to adapt rapidly to changed surroundings.[13]

Another answer for obesity by the 1990s came to be bariatric surgery. Genetic information about obesity (or any other pathological state) had not led in any cases to new therapies; so older therapeutic means became newly fashionable. The first surgeries, jejunoileal bypasses, were performed in the 1950s at the University of Minnesota, intentionally to cause malabsorption by bypassing most of the intestines and causing weight loss. This surgery performed detached all but 12 in. to 18 in. of the small bowel and set it to the side. But the uncontrolled malabsorption of nutrients that resulted almost always led to severe negative health consequences. In the late 1960s Drs. Edward Mason and Chikashi Ito developed the gastric bypass at the University of Iowa. In the late 1970s, Dr. Ward Griffin refined the gastric bypass into its currently most popular form, the Roux-en-Y (RYGBP). This surgically bypasses most of the stomach and a small amount of the small intestine to limit the amount of nutrition actually absorbed. All procedures were available to treat obesity and once it was claimed that obesity was heavily genetically determined, it was assumed that only such radical cures would override the genetic code.

However, in 1997, researchers presented a claim that obesity could be caused in part by an infectious agent, adenovirus Ad-36. Nikhil Dhurandhar and Richard Atkinson undertook to show that, "This increase [in obesity] is the type of pattern that might occur with a new infectious disease, as has been seen with the AIDS virus."[14] Obesity was not genetic as its epidemiology in the United States showed that it was concentrated in those states with massive chicken production. And chickens spread the Ad-36 virus. (Researchers had raised this claim in 1960s only to abandon this line of inquiry.) So perhaps surgery is not the answer, but rather the development, as with HIV and AIDS, of a new obesity vaccine?

Dhurandhar noted that such a pattern of infection may well solve the mystery of the rapid spread of

> ...obesity [which] has been called the number one public health problem in America. The etiology of obesity is considered to be multifactorial...While genetic and behavioral components of obesity have been the focus of intense study, an infection as an etiological factor has received little attention. Although "infectobesity," a new term to describe obesity of infectious origin, appears to be a new concept, over the past twenty years, six different pathogens have been reported to cause obesity in animal models. The relative contribution of these pathogens to human obesity is unknown.[15]

Such an anti-viral agent would simply "cure" obesity. "In 10 years," Dhurandhar stated in an interview, "people may be able to walk into a clinic and be told that their obesity is due to X cause, such as genes, the endocrine system, or pathogens. That may have a more productive outcome than a blanket treatment right now, [which] is not very successful. And because viruses are hard or impossible to treat, prevention through vaccines will be key."[16]

These claims were based on decades of research. As early as the 1970s, Dhurandhar had observed that a chicken adeno-virus, isolated in Bombay, caused chickens to accumulate as much as 50% more fat than healthy birds. The virus also lowered the animals' cholesterol and triglyceride levels before it killed them. What interested him at that time though was the odd fact that infected chickens ate no more than uninfected ones. Dhurandhar and his colleagues identified the infectious agents as Ad-36. This agent was first isolated in humans in 1978 in the fecal matter of a 7-year-old diabetic girl.

Inspired by the discovery of Ad-36, Dhurandhar began to theorize that it might be a contributing factor to the skyrock-eting obesity epidemic in human beings. He next looked for evidence of infection with the chicken virus in a group of fifty-two obese people. Ten showed signs of infection; there-fore, it was an avian-spread virus that was postulated as the cause, a "bird-flu" model that might spread to human beings. Commentators also responded immediately to the "possibility that obesity is a viral disease." Some argued that Ad-36 had serious social consequences as, "It may give people ammuni-tion to fight for insurance coverage for weight-loss treatment because they could argue: 'I've got a reason. I'm not just a fat slob.'"[17] The claim that obesity was simply a public sign of the lack of willpower, one of the most powerful notions driving older images about obesity, could finally be stilled by the very notion that its cause was beyond the individual (and even beyond the individual's genetic make-up) and was to be found in the ever more dangerous world of infectious diseases. It could also help explain the odd demographics of the "obesity epidemic" as it moved from the coasts and then toward the midsection of the USA, that is from areas of intense chicken farming to areas that have far fewer chickens.

While clearly important, Dhurandhar's research was not the first attempt to define obesity as the symptom of an infectious disease. The noted Rockefeller University geneticist, Jules Hirsch, attempted to do so very early in his career. In a 1982 paper, he and his colleagues found "An obesity syndrome…in a number of mice infected as young adults with canine distemper virus, a morbillivirus antigenically related to measles." These mice, according to Hirsch, had more and larger fat cells than their uninfected littermates. The researchers thought that the infections might well have altered brain pathways to encourage cell alteration and growth. No "natural" (genetic) process here but rather a response to a pathological agent.[18] This trajectory, however, was quickly abandoned for a "genetically" determined hypothesis for the existence of obesity.

For all of the desire to stop the image of the obese being at fault for their own misery, the idea of infectobesity provided yet one more level to the anxiety about the obesity epidemic. Here is an additional force through which to imagine how the fear attendant to the very notion of infectious diseases can be used to focus and define a moral panic that may well have only a tangential relationship to the very notion of infection itself. What is remarkable about the notion of infectious diseases in the age of AIDS is that it couples the idea of the origin of disease in a distant foreign place with the fear of an uncontrolled

spread answered almost simultaneously with the announce-
ment of a cure, a quick fix or magic bullet.

Some explanations for obesity, such as infections, imply
intervention and cure. Yet genetic explanations seem to deny
(at least today) any form of intervention and treatment. There
are over forty different complex syndromes listed in the on-line
"Mendelian Inheritance in Man" database that include "obesity"
as one of the diagnostic criteria. Yet each may well trigger
different combinations of genes for different reasons. The
discovery of these and other hormones could provide a scientific basis to treat individuals who have high body fat in the
same way that doctors treat high blood pressure or cholesterol.
Furthermore, such genetic anomalies could also be detected
by genetic screening in analogy to Downs Syndrome and identify high-risk individuals.

Such approaches are counter indicators to massive interventions in social planning, such as high taxes on foods seen as the
cause of obesity, that have been suggested in the UK and the
USA. Foods labeled "unhealthy" and seen as contributing to
obesity should be taxed as tobacco and alcohol are now taxed.
The "fat tax" would make unhealthy food more expensive with
the hope of compelling people to make healthier diet choices.
A cure for "weakness of the will" but perhaps not a cure for the
genetically predisposed to obesity or those exposed to a virus
that might cause obesity.

The consensus at the close of the twentieth century was that
obesity was a major health problem and that obese individuals
were the production of a misalignment between their genetics
and the world they inhabited. One social product of the stigmatization of the obese by the 1960s was the appearance of
advocacy groups of overweight individuals who argued not

only that their bodily status should not be stigmatized but also that they were happy and proud to be fat. This complete reversal of the medicalization of obesity resuscitated the earlier claim that Kim Chernin had made that we all live in a world dominated by a "tyranny of slenderness."

The NAAFA (originally the National Association to Aid Fat Americans, later changed to National Association to Advance Fat Acceptance) was founded in 1969 to "eliminate discrimination based on body size and provide fat people with the tools for self-empowerment through public education, advocacy, and member support."[9] It splintered in 1973 and members of the Los Angeles chapter founded the Fat Underground, a collective of fat activists with strong ties to the radical therapy, lesbian, and feminist communities. They published the "Fat Liberation Manifesto," a document outlining the collective's political ties to other oppressed and minority groups, its anti-diet stance, and its demand for equality in all areas of life for fat women. They argue, as does the International Size Acceptance Association (ISAA), that a person can be healthy at any size. They condemn the use of fear, guilt, and misinformation by the diet industry to sell (at best useless and at worst dangerous) products to consumers of all sizes. In their official position statement on dieting and the diet industry, the NAAFA emphasizes that the suffering of fat people is due to the stereotypes perpetuated by the diet industry as well as the world of medicine. The various permutations of NAAFA, such as the Chicago Size Acceptance Group, have turned the tables; it is claimed, on the claims of the medicalization of obesity by allowing overweight individuals to take pride in their size.

Thus the struggle over who are fat and why they are fat, and the question of whether obesity is a natural state or a disease process continues. While the science of obesity has provided new insights into the mechanisms by which weight is maintained and increased, the meanings associated with overweight continue to be contested as the struggle over the fat body comes to dominate the headlines of our daily newspapers and the concerns of the national and international public health communities.

VII

THE "ORIENT" BATTLES OBESITY

U p to this point in our history of obesity we have looked at Western models of obesity. There is an alternative tale: that of Chinese medicine and how it adopts the rhetoric of obesity from Western medicine. In Shigehisa Kuriyama's *The Expressiveness of the Body and the Divergence of Greek and Chinese Medicine* (1999), the standard study of ancient Greek and traditional Chinese medicine, the "model" body type in classical Chinese literature is described as rotund, as opposed to the muscular and svelte men of Greek art. Obesity seems not to be a problem in the various theories of the ill body in Chinese medicine. Yet with the modernization of China during the late nineteenth century, the question of obesity enters into allopathic as well as traditional medicine. At the end of the Empire, Western medical missionaries viewed China as a famine society. The modernizing tendencies in Republican China see just the opposite: China is a world at risk from obesity. Obesity is a sign both of the degeneracy of the Imperial past as well as of modernity and its treatments need to be those imported from the West. At the start of the twenty-first century the medical establishment in the People's Republic

130

of China again sees obesity as a major public health threat, which is a sign of the Westernization of Chinese society. It is McDonald's that weakens the will of the Chinese people through advertizing. Childhood obesity in contemporary China is seen as the result of globalization, that is, of Americanization: it is Ronald McDonald who is at fault. The public health establishment sees the rejection of industrialized ("fast") food as a cure but also imports everything from "fat camps" to theories about ethnic predisposition to obesity from the West. China has become a world where modern obesity is medicalized and treated in ways that echo as well as blame Western society.

Recent studies of obesity in China have come to reverse the claim that such food-borne diseases invade from the primitive "Orient." These Chinese-based studies are often rooted in the view that obesity and its attendant symptoms are the result of the recent pathological "Occidentalization" of China and the Chinese. This obsession with the "contamination from the West" has come to be part of the explanation of obesity in contemporary medicine in China (the People's Republic) as well as Western medicine dealing with the Diaspora Chinese.

In early twentieth-century China there was a popular fascination with obesity, perhaps as a result of the images of "famine" that marked Western views of the pathological body in nineteenth-century China. When you systematically read the standard "Western" medical journal published in China, the *China Medical Journal*, from the beginning of the twentieth century to the Japanese invasion of China, the central medical discourse concerning "diet" and the body is that of famine and starvation. The physicians of the China Medical Missionary Association are concerned that the food made available in their hospitals has sufficient protein and fat, to the extent that they advocate "crossing foreign and native cows," or the introduction of canned milk to improve the local diet.[1] That diet seems to be regionally differentiated. One physician notes that the "rich have rice, vegetables, and meats. The poor have rice, vegetables and substitutes for meat." It is only "when floods overtake the people year in and year out that so many are driven to our doors for charity."[2] China is, from this perspective, not a "famine" culture at all. Rather it is the distribution of foods that seem to be at the heart of famine from the standpoint of the physicians. In this rather contemporary view it is the distribution network that causes famine.[3] (Amartya Sen's 1981 *Poverty and Famines: An Essay on Entitlement and Deprivation* argues that famine occurs not from a lack of food, but from inequalities built into mechanisms for distributing food.) But there is also some suspicion that the indigenous foods may not be "suitable" enough to maintain a healthy diet.[4] The soybean is advocated over and over again as adequate as a substitute for other forms of protein.[5]

Yet when the concern is true starvation the sense is that "Western" cures, such as a rich, milk-based diet is most appropriate.[6] It is the child who is seen as most at risk from the effects of famine. The selling of children is seen as a major result of the famine culture of China.[7] "Cannot the famine relief associations...take this matter into consideration and put an end to it," writes one irate physician.[8] In all of the myriad concerns about the pathological effects of diet, not a single word is spent about the dangers or effects of obesity.[9]

The concern with obesity appears in Chinese popular magazines, where it is already seen as a response to the past and the contemporary, allopathic-medicine view of China as a famine

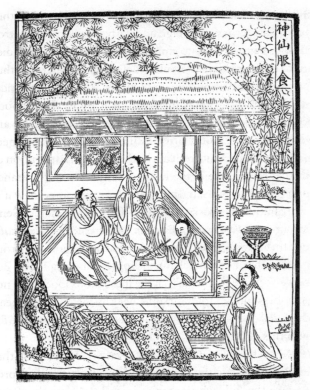

16. Two men sitting in a hall, earnestly discussing dietetic methods of achieving longevity during the Ming period (1368–1644). On the right, a child is kneeling on the floor, stirring a concoction simmering over a furnace. The diet of the Immortals (*shenxian fushi*) was the name given to one of the four genres of ancient Chinese medical literature. (*Wellcome Collection*)

culture. This is not to say that there has not been a constant and intense concern with the "immoderate body" in the medical and dietetic literature of traditional Chinese medicine. In the sixteenth century Li Shizhen (1518–93) wrote in his *Bencai gangmu* (*Systematic Materia Medica*) that the consumption of fresh crabs was healthy "in small quantities" but, "Gluttons will consume a dozen or more at a sitting together with various kinds of meat and other foods. They eat and drink twice as much as they need...then blame [their upset stomachs on] the crabs. But why blame the crabs?"[10] The culture of excess in the world of traditional Chinese medicine became a hallmark of the degenerate Chinese body in need of regeneration by the early twentieth century. From a Western perspective it was the result of the political system that had made China into the "sick man of Asia": "Apoplexy among the aged officials in Peking, properly disposed to it by their obesity and their having to perform the nine obeisances before the emperor so frequently, is not very uncommon."[11] Or perhaps it was because of the Imperial cultural practices that encouraged endogenous marriages:

> The whole race displays a remarkable tendency to obesity. The nutritious juices of the body are directed toward the surface distending and overloading the cellular tissues with inordinate quantity of fat. This general tendency of the whole people can only be attributed to the hereditary diathesis unchecked by intermarriage with others differently constituted. It is an evil which exclusiveness of that singular people has entailed upon them.[12]

But if this is the case at least, unlike other "obese" peoples, they were spared the curse of diabetes, which "is said to be very uncommon in China and Japan."[13] But in all cases this is the result of change over time as, "One gets the impression that most Chinese babies are born with excellent health and are particularly round and fat and chubby and though congenital deformities are not uncommonly met with, congenital disease is comparatively rarely so."[14] It is cultural practice that causes healthy, "chubby" babies to become obese adults.

Such claims were quite in contrast to the anxiety about emaciation, which drove thin people to undertake "special bulking diets" in order to find marriage partners. Such emaciation was often seen as the curse of ancestors who were "'eating' the health and vitality of a descendant in retaliation for neglect or mistreatment. Plumpness, by contrast, was perceived as a clear indication that the person so blessed was in harmony with the supernatural world."[15] Yet this dominant image of China as a starvation culture had its answer in the counter example of the degenerate obese body, also present in the world of early twentieth-century China.

Immediately before the revolution that overthrew the Qing dynasty on October 10, 1911, "reform" was everywhere. A new fantasy of the "reformed" body had begun to emerge in China. Obesity came to be viewed as one of the signs of the degenerate Chinese body, a body clearly in need of reform, because of the excesses of Imperial China and the exploitation of the "sick man of Asia" by colonial powers. Following the model of "regeneration" that captured most of the ideologies of the day (from Zionism to Marxism to Social Darwinism to Colonialism), obesity defines the ability of the new society to reform the individual and his or her body. In one of the most widely read columns, "Ziyoutan" ("unfettered talk"), in the renowned newspaper *Shenbao*, the author Wang Dungen explored the reform of the body. He was a well-known writer who was a key figure in the "Mandarin Ducks and Butterflies School." Wang Dungen was attacked by the May Fourth progressive writers in the late 1910s and early 1920s, and in 1914 created the comic journal *Saturday*. In this comic essay, "Reforming the Human Body," Wang Dungen envisions a grotesque ideal of the "new" body. He imagines a body with newly configured mouth, tongue, ear, eyes, nose, skin, eyebrow, hair, teeth, neck, shoulders, arm, hands, fingers, and feet. He sees it as having hundreds of mouths so that a person can eat more and still be able to talk.[16] This is an ironic response to the starved body, which desires a reform that can permit it to consume ever more. "Western" models of regeneration, such as structured physical exercise, become the means of reforming the too fat body. Chen Duxiu, the leader of the New Cultural Movement, advocated exercise to make the Chinese physically as well as morally fit, and Mao Zedong in 1917 published a full-scale manual of physical activity to reform the body.[17]

By 1913 the new medical literature on obesity was beginning to be summarized for an intellectual readership in China. The essay "On Obesity," by Shuhui and Weiseng, was written in classical Chinese for a leading women's magazine. Such magazines arose to shape and be shaped by the images of the so-called New Woman (xin nuxing) and Westernized Modern Girl (modeng nulang) who came into prominence in the first decade of the twentieth century in China as well as in the West. They were defined in many ways, to no little extent by their "thin" body form. Thinness, even after the establishment of the People's Republic, as James L. Watson noted, continued to be a mark of "bad luck, illness, and early death."[18] It was the "stigma of emaciation" that scarred the psyche of the Chinese at the beginning and the close of the twentieth century. However, it was associated not with "modern" thought, but with village superstition and backwardness among the intellectuals of the early twentieth century.

The essay of 1913 presents the argument that obesity is an illness that women must not take lightly.[19] The authors refer to male figures and texts from ancient China, such as a man named "Zilong" who lived in the Warring States period from 476 BCE to the unification of China by the Qin Dynasty in 221 BCE. Zilong felt that he was too fat, so he took *Phragmites communis Trirn* (a traditional medicine) to lose weight. The authors use this example to prove that obesity was an illness treatable by medical intervention even in the pre-modern period. One source they mention is *Hanshu* (*The History of the Former Han Dynasty*), written by the historian Bangu. They argue that according to Hanshu, too much body fat is the cause of obesity. But there are two kinds of obesity; one is obesity with too many blood cells and the other not enough blood cells. The causes of the former are not eating appropriately, not having a balanced lifestyle, and not enough sex. Not eating appropriately means that one eats too many unhealthy foods, such as flour, sugar, and alcohol. Obesity of the second type is caused by external injury, overworking, stress, or sometimes after giving birth.

As with the Western literature of the late nineteenth century, there are stages of obesity.[20] For the authors, obesity has three phases. Initially, the person looks acceptably plump, which indicates prosperity so that others admire him; then he looks overtly obese and funny; and, finally, he is in danger and others take pity on him. This final stage of obesity presents many symptoms including sweating, fatigue, backache, heart disease, and sexual incompetence. The "cure" for obesity is balanced eating and lifestyle: avoid eating things that contain too much fat, don't sleep more than eight hours, take a warm bath two or three times a week, walk two or three hours every day, and be persistent. In terms of medication, one should take either traditional medication, such as *wodu*, or, better yet, thyroid tablets. The latter were the newest pharmaceutical intervention and certainly can reduce weight by making the individual hyper-thyroidal, which increases basal metabolism. This will lead to weight loss but can lead to a wide range of other pathologies of hyperthyroidism. The argument here is that there is a Chinese traditional manner of treating obesity that is parallel to the most modern, Western medical interventions. The degeneration of the end of the Imperial period, with its excesses, is bracketed by an older medical tradition as well as a modern one that can deal with the results of such excesses.

The modern creeps into this world of classical Chinese views on the obese with the suggestion of treating it as an endocrino-logical deficiency, one of the most up-to-date views in early twentieth-century medicine. For while the obese body is always defined as the antithesis of the beautiful and healthy body, this is a special problem for contemporary women. In an essay, "Keep the Body Slim," published in a women's magazine in 1922, the author, Daizuo, stresses that people with obesity are not beautiful, especially women: "A person who is too fat looks very ugly. Women especially can't be fat. If a woman gains too much weight and becomes fatty, where can one find her beauty?"[21] In addition, obesity is an important medical problem. Obesity is seen as the result of faulty metabolism, the result of hormone imbalance. Yet obesity is not a random occurrence as some people are more at risk. Specifically, people who eat rich and abundant food, people who are not physically active, people with a family inheritance of obesity, and alco-holics.

Obesity is dangerous as it leads to heart disease. People with obesity have shortness of breath and rapid heartbeats even after walking a few steps. They are more likely to have strokes. People with obesity have urinary and kidney problems. Dieting is again the solution. One should not overeat; one should avoid food that contains too much fat and eat less meat. Other suggestions the essay gives for weight loss are physical exercises, the use of laxatives, and electric steam therapy to reduce body fat, which according to the essay is very popular abroad. As we have discussed earlier in this book, electrotherapy was a standard late-nineteenth-century Western treatment for the "failure or perversion of nutrition," including diabetes.[22]

Women were clearly the target of the growing anti-obesity anxiety of Republican China. In one essay, the author, Zhou Zhenyu, states that he is a doctor who often has female patients who need help to lose weight.[23] Zhou Zhenyu comments, "When I was a doctor in Beiping, I often had women patients come asking for the method of losing weight. I would tell them the method, some of them went home and practiced following my suggestions, others would come visit again and want medication. The effects differ because the causes of their obesity vary." "The cause and danger of female obesity" is seen either in overindulgence and the absence of exercise or imbalance of hormones. This is the classic argument about obesity that dominated the late-nineteenth-century discussion of the causes of obesity. In the United States, by 1924, the home of most of the medical missionaries in China, the editors of the *Journal of the American Medical Association* had published an editorial entitled "What Causes Obesity?" In it they argue, following a powerful anti-psychological strand in obesity research that began in the late nineteenth century, for its etiology in malfunctions of normal metabolic processes. See obesity as a "scientific problem," they write, and that will free the "fat woman" from the stigma that she "has the remedy in her own hands—or rather between her own teeth." The new object of scientific interest is the fat woman, who had been charged with carrying "that extra weight about with her unless she so wills."[24] Women, not "men" or "people" were at risk from obesity, a far cry from the evocation of Dickens' "Fat Boy" as the exemplary sufferer from obesity in the mid-nineteenth century. According to an anonymous Chinese physician in 1922, although fat people usually eat less than thin people, they do not burn enough calories. There are still large amounts of fat accumulated and stored in their body. While the obese do not eat much every meal, they snack often. Women specifically can suffer from hypothyroidism, hypopituitarism, or a loss of estrogen. Pregnant women are especially at risk. One woman, after giving birth, had to get up and eat every night. She quickly gained weight and became obese.

The danger of female obesity is the collapse of one's health and thus one's ability to bear children. This remains the classic definition of women's health. Obese women have compromised immune systems, are likely to catch cold and coughs, which leads to tuberculosis. They have heart disease. There is danger to one's nervous system. The obese are usually slow and lazy, but oftentimes they laugh and seem happy. Obese women have problems conceiving, have problems when having sex, and are likely to have miscarriages.

By 1941, as the war raged and famine haunted China, a public discourse on obesity remained part of the popular register of the new "reformed" Chinese attitude toward the body. These attitudes came to be labeled as a "tragedy at the dinner table." An essay of this title[25] seems to be a free adaptation of a number of foreign medical and popular articles, especially American ones. It presents the pathological consequences of overeating. The author identifies middle-aged people as most at risk, because they seem to be more easily taken by the desire for fine eating. The essay defines pathology by quoting a saying attributed to an American congressman: "fifty, fifty, fifty," which means that if a 50-year-old person is 50 lb. (3 stones 8 lb.) overweight, his life span will be reduced by 50%. The author also quotes statistics by an American doctor that out of 2,000 cases of sudden death, 90% people died of heart disease. "Most of them eat too much, are overweight, which causes heart disease." While other foreign cases of overeating are mentioned, such as the ancient Romans, the American Thanksgiving Day is picked out as a moment of public gluttony:

> Around Thanksgiving time, there are often cases of death caused by overeating to be found in the mortuary. People in charge of the post-mortem examinations are often too busy rushing to luxurious banquets to do their work. It's also quite dangerous to eat too much after fasting. One should definitely divide all the nice dishes into several meals, and never eat everything at once. It is nice to be able to enjoy a full table of luxurious food, but one should remember not to gamble with one's own life. Otherwise tragedy would take place in the holiday season, and one would sadly fall onto the bosom of the death.

The result of such gluttony is sudden death, chronic heart disease, or diabetes. A litany of diseases is the result of obesity: high blood pressure, lung disease, cancer, even suicide and accidental death. For, according to the author, people with obesity often have psychological problems and are very slow in reacting to what is going on—thus becoming prone to accidents. The overweight should consult qualified doctors to decide his or her individual diet. Yet the "cure" proposed in the essay of 1941 is to pay minute attention to what and how much one eats. The formula does not have much to do with any specific type of food; rather that as one gets older, one should eat less. When one gets very old, one should only eat light and simple food, returning to the diet prescribed for infants.

The fear of obesity has reappeared in China during the past decade among a generation that sees famine as being a thing of the past. This generation, at the beginning of the twenty-first century, now sees itself as a culture of excess in response to the memories and tales of famine told by its parents and grandparents. James L. Watson noted that the dominant sense of fear concerning the body in modern China is the result of the great famine under Mao Zedong.[26] This famine, from 1958 to 1961, which resulted from the collectivization of the peasants killed millions in China and evoked the horrors of the famines of the 1940s during the war against the Japanese, the civil war, and the policies of the nationalist government. For adults in today's China, "famine" evokes their own experiences after Mao as well as the tales of starvation by their parents and grandparents.

Yet the concern with obesity appears at the close of the twentieth century. In a retrospective analysis of a detailed, nationwide survey of illnesses ascribed to dietary causes in the 1980s and 1990s, obesity was hardly mentioned, except to note that "obesity was a much less central concern in China."[27] In the twenty-first century the "obesity epidemic" seems to be the next great fear of Chinese public health officers following smoking: "Chronic diseases now account for an estimated 80% of deaths and 70% of disability-adjusted life-years lost in China. Cardiovascular diseases and cancer are the leading causes of both death and the burden of disease, and exposure to risk factors is high: more than 300 million men smoke cigarettes and 160 million adults are hypertensive, most of whom are not being treated. An obesity epidemic is imminent, with more than 20% of children aged 7–17 years in big cities now overweight or obese."[28] Childhood in the twenty-first century means being at risk. The transition, from smoking to obesity as the most important threat to public health clearly parallels the fear in Western sources, such as the World Health Organization, that had identified obesity as the next great danger—having "eliminated" smoking as a public health hazard.

For China, with an increasing number of people now smoking, and where tobacco remains a major source of state revenue, obesity is the new danger. The fat child, not the Marlboro Man, is the source of anxiety. Smoking is popularly seen as a "positive" reflection of the process of modernization, while obesity has come to represent the corruption imported from the West. The official journal of "preventive medicine," *Zhonghua Yu Fang Yi Xue Za Zhi*, acknowledged in 2005 that "The prevalence of overweight and obesity among people living in rural areas was lower than that of their urban counterparts ... It was estimated that another 70 million overweight and 30 million obese Chinese people emerged in China from 1992 to 2002. The prevalence of overweight and obesity of Chinese people has increased rapidly in the past decade, which had affected 260 million Chinese people. It would continue to increase in the near future if effective intervention measures were not taken."[29] The shift seems to be marked. A body mass index of greater than $25 \, \text{kg/m}^2$ is to be found in 18.7% of the population in urban areas as opposed to 13.7% in rural areas. (We should note that a BMI of 30 is conventionally held to be obese.) But the increase over the past decades is also striking. These figures are for 1997. They mark a fourfold increase over

1982, when only 3.7% of Chinese adults had a BMI of over 25.[30] Chinese medical and epidemiological studies argue that "Obesity has become a global epidemic," though there seems to be little knowledge of the state of affairs in China (meaning the People's Republic of China). Looking at "a group of 2,776 randomly selected adults (20–94 years of age) living in the Huayang Community in Shanghai, China," this 2002 study argued that while "the prevalence of obesity" [using Western standards] was lower in China than in the West, the "overall fat mass-related metabolic disorders were also common."[31] The Chinese, unlike the Japanese, seem to have been growing "fat" over the past fifty years without developing greater height or frame size. Rather than the positive aspects of a change in diet being measured, only the pathological results of overweight preoccupy the medical scientists. Thus the diseases of "modernity" such as diabetes are often the proof of a decaying, decadent population, just as it was in the nineteenth century in studies of diabetes. Today the argument is that diabetes is more than twice as frequent in the Chinese (urban) overweight population, even though this population is overall of lower weight than the equivalent Western population. The visible pathology of obesity was immediately translated into the invisible disease of diabetes. But what is the cause?

Westernization and "economic success" in the new China or among Diaspora Chinese is seen as the ultimate cause of the disease. The urbanization of China is read as the source of both shifts in patterns of food consumption as well as changes in work habits. Both lead to what is now called "metabolic syndromes," the diseases associated with obesity.[32] All of these shifts are read as aspects of "Americanization," the new cause of obesity. America is now the source of illness rather than, as in the early twentieth century, the place from where "cure" may come.[33] James L. Watson noted that McDonald's is the test case for the positive or negative implications of "Yankee imperialism."[34] Or, as he points out in the 2006 update to his book on "fast food" in China, McDonald's has become paradigmatic of the new evil: globalization.[35] Yet in the eyes of the Chinese authorities and the public, McDonald's represented "modernization, hygiene, and responsible management."[36] In a complex way, it represented a healthy food as opposed to the traditional "street food," which was seen as dangerous. McDonald's represented the "invention of cleanliness" in Hong Kong and beyond.[37] In Taipei, McDonald's was actually credited with "promoting hygiene and etiquette." A school principal there observed, "Every set lunch is wrapped in a clean bag. Students become accustomed to using a napkin during meals. They learn hygienic behavior and proper etiquette by eating hamburgers."[38] Today McDonald's represents the intrusion of a "homogenous, global culture." But this is also a hygienic culture because of its emphasis on its homogeneity in what is seen as a chaotic "Chinese" food culture, which is imagined as posing health risks.

The medical readings of such changes were, however, solely negative, and had little to do with improved food safety. Tsung O. Cheng of George Washington University's medical school has made the claim concerning even the recent work on obesity in China that "the proportion of obesity among children under the age of 15 increased from 15% in 1982 to 27% today" because of "fast food and physical inactivity." "All of the children in China recognize the image of Ronald McDonald, even though they may not be able to read English."[39] Zumin Shi of the Jiangsu Provincial Center for Disease Control and Prevention looks at the expansion of obesity-related illnesses such as anemia among adolescents in the new China and correlates this with parental attention and "overnutrition".[40] J. X. Jiang at the National Center for Women's and Children's Health examines a similar problem in terms of family structure for the etiology and intervention of obesity.[41] Bin Xie, a social worker who is based in California looks at data from Wuhan to correlate mental state (depression) and obesity among the newly successful who now lack an adequate social network. The claim is that "the findings of this study may contribute to our understanding of the influences of psychological correlates in pediatric overweight in the Eastern cultural environment."[42] All imagine that obesity is a reflex of the altered status of individual, family, and society with the most recent changes in the economic system. Yet there is also a compelling counterview: that the changes in the weight of immigrants tend not to shift greatly when they come to the United States.[43] The view seems to be that America provides all the wrong incentives; only traditional values (and diet) preserve health.

What happens when we leave (for a moment) China and move with the Chinese Diaspora to that land of McDonald's, America? Jyu-Lin Chen and Christine Kennedy examine correlative material in an analysis of overweight Chinese-American children that suggests "that a more democratic parenting style contributes to a higher BMI in Chinese-American children. First, several studies have shown that an authoritarian parenting style in Chinese families may not necessarily reflect the strict parenting that was measured in Western society. Conversely, parents' involvement, care, supervision, and encouragement of academic achievement, all of which typically have been identified as components of an "authoritarian" parenting style in

Western society, are, in fact, a reflection of caring and loving parenting in the Chinese culture."[44] American-type success breaks down the "parental control and warmth" that constitutes Chinese child raising and leads to fat Chinese children who are a pathological sign of that success: "A democratic parenting style and poor family communication contribute to higher BMI in Chinese-American children."[45] All obesity comes from the West. Chinese families, understood as a traditional society (certainly not in terms of the Cultural Revolution), simply don't produce fat kids. Only children raised in the traditional "Chinese" manner (not children raised in the American manner) are not at risk, unless, of course, they live in Shanghai.

There are, of course, large numbers of "Asian-Americans" who fall below the poverty line. They are seen to be at risk of the obesity associated in contemporary medical argument with poverty. In this way too they mimic "typical" American dietary patterns. In one study, "Asian-American ethnic groups," defined as the Chinese, Vietnamese, and Hmong in California, were the focus. In this study, "The concept of good health [in these communities] included having a harmonious family, balance, and mental and emotional stability. All groups also expressed the general belief that specific foods have hot or cold properties and are part of the Yin–Yang belief system common to Asian cultures. The lure of fast food, children's adoption of American eating habits, and long work hours were identified as barriers to a healthy, more traditional lifestyle."[46] Yet the results here are virtually identical with those whose belief systems were very different. All classify the "poor" as those at risk for the pathologies of obesity. In fact, one recent study has argued that children in China stunted by malnutrition are at substantially greater risk from obesity as they mature.[47]

"America" serves as more than the place where obesity has its origin. In many Chinese studies, the model of a multiethnic America, with different rates of risk, becomes the model for understanding different groups' responses to obesity. What was once a monolithic risk to the "Chinese" becomes a more differentiated risk, where ethnic subgroups are seen as at greater risk because of their implied genetic or cultural differences. Looking at "ethnic" populations in Xinjiang, a recent study documented that more "obese" Kazak people developed hypertension, whereas more "obese" Uygur people developed diabetes. Implicitly the difference in "genetic" background was suggested as the cause, using American studies of African-American and Mexican-American obesity and the resultant increase in cases of type II diabetes in these communities. (The People's Republic of China includes fifty-six national minorities but the "majority" Han is itself a composite category.) It is also clear that the Uygur subjects were from rural south Xinjiang and the Kazak subjects from suburban north Xinjiang.[48] Thus the "Han" become the unspoken parallel to the labels in American majority culture: epidemiologically rarely differentiated and labeled "white" or "Caucasian." This is just as constructed a "majority" category in opposition to the other minority and therefore "racial" ones, as is the Han.[49] This is a subset of the construction of the "yellow race," which, according to Jing Tsu, is one of the formative myths of modern Chinese identity.[50] Each such construction seeks out some category, which is at risk of stressing the "healthy" nature of the racial category seen as dominant. In the nineteenth century, it was the "healthy" German Jew as opposed to the sickly Eastern Jew. The "rural versus urban" question of healthy versus unhealthy "ethnicities" replicates this dichotomy. They are here as muddy as those studies of obesity in the developed world that seem to reveal that for ethnic minorities, as in the West, ethnicity trumps geography (or rather biology trumps class). Indeed, there is even the argument that urban sprawl does not impact on weight, rather that fat people "choose to live in more sprawling neighbour-hoods" as opposed to "mixed use" ones as they would rather get about by car than walk.[51]

But we need to ask if "obesity" in "Asia" is the same phenom-enological category as in the "West"? Not only are there different histories of the "large" body and its meaning in "Asia" but there are different physiological measures that would be used for the definition of the obese body. I use the label "Asia" in this context rather than "Chinese" as in 2002 The World Health Organization called a meeting in Hong Kong to examine whether the obese body was to be defined differently among "Asians." This "led to the proposal that adult over-weight could be specified in Asia when the body mass index exceeded 23.00 and obesity should be specified when the BMI exceed 25.00."[52] This is substantially (almost ten points) lower than the American criteria, which should include that new category "Asian-Americans." Yet it is clear that the Asian-American population is being measured by Western public health definitions of overweight and obesity. What are the boundaries of "Asia"? Do they now contain Taiwan, which sees itself in the context of the Pacific islands? Does Asia reach north into Mongolia and Siberia? To the Ainu? To the West to India? Or is it a composite that rests in an American fantasy of the "Asian"? Bodily changes among Japanese-Americans over three generations after immigration have been demonstrated. Yet there seems to be no increase in obesity except over the past decade, with the imposition of "Western" definitions of "obesity."[53] Indeed, "Japanese Women don't get Old or Fat," according to the title of a recent book that claims that Japan has the lowest obesity rate in the developed world, the longest life expenditure, and the lowest per capita health care cost.[54] It postulates a "Japanese Paradox" (analogous to the "French paradox" and the claim of universal thinness in France): "How can the world's most food-obsessed nation have the lowest obesity rates in the industrialized world—and the best longevity on Earth? The answer given is diet: "The Asian diet is probably the best on earth."[55] Yet the takeaway foods available are Western: "Italian, Chinese, French, and Indian, since food in Japan has been a global affair for many centuries."[56] "Sushi" (as well as McDonald's and pizza) has gone global since it was first mentioned in the *Ladies' Home Journal* in 1929 as not sounding quite as delicious as it is to the untutored reader.[57] The sushi craze does not seem to have altered the American sense of what are healthful foods, even at the glatt kosher Shalom Sushi, a New York restaurant playing to two contemporary senses of what is healthy food. Health promotion, as Richard Parish has noted, is a concept not much older than the 1980s.[58] In that light, "Japanese" food comes, along with "kosher" food to be read as inherently "healthful" even though such claims are rarely made for it at its point of origin.

No such claims are made about the low impact of Western foods, such as pizza and curry, on China. A recent popular American study claims that the Chinese diet is the answer to Western obesity.[59] Its authors stress that the "difference between rural Chinese diets and Western diets, and the ensuing disease patterns, is enormous."[60] Their claim is that "cancer" is primarily the result of the ingestion of animal fats. For them the paucity of such fats in the traditional Chinese diet may explain the different epidemiology of cancer in contemporary China. There is nostalgia for the food that "natural man," living in harmony with nature, consumed which protected him from the diseases of modernity, such as obesity. Indeed even a recent, more serious epidemiological study of the shifts in Chinese eating and work patterns and their proposed impact on weight gain begins with the statement: "The classic Chinese diet based on rice and vegetables is being replaced by increasing amounts of animal products and a Western-type diet profile."[61] The inhabitants of northern China, with their heavily meat (pork) oriented diets would clearly take exception to the creation of a "classic Chinese diet" that seems to reflect a Western homogenization of the wide range of cuisines that exist and existed throughout the broadest reaches of what is now called China. That there is a change in eating patterns may well be the case: but the creation of an ideal Chinese diet belies both the diversity of Chinese eating patterns and the existence of rural famine even in areas that do reflect such a reliance on "rice and vegetables."

Westernization in both China and the Chinese Diaspora may well play a role but it is a secondary cause—the primary cause is the long established one-child policy in China and the change in the status of urban children. This change is analogous to the attitudes of many first-generation immigrants in the American urban Diaspora (not only the Chinese). Yet a preoccupation with the diseases of obesity, specifically diabetes (type II) is found within this literature on China. In a paper from 2001, a study of adults in a population of northeastern China, specifically in Da Qing City argued, "Increasing waist measurements predicted tenfold increases in hypertension and a three-to-five times increased risk of diabetes. Suitable waist cut-off points were 85 cm for men and 80 cm for women, with statistical analysis showing waist circumference as the more dominant predictor of risk than age, waist-to-hip ratios, or BMIs. Hence, small increases in BMI, and particularly in waist circumference, predict a substantial increase in the risk of diabetes...in Chinese adults."[62] What is being seen is a shift in body size because of the accessibility of different foods. What may be being observed is the so-called "thrifty genotype" hypothesis that had been suggested in 1964. When one thus measured first generation groups of immigrants to the United States in the late nineteenth century, there was a substantially lower rate of diabetes. The initial groups showed an extremely low index of obesity and the resultant diabetes. This index, however, skyrocketed after just a short time of living in their new environment. Thus, as mentioned before, diabetes and obesity seem to be an index of a failure to adapt rapidly to changed surroundings. It is the rapidity of change that lies at the heart of the matter.

In China today, rural children are suffering from malnutrition. The Beijing-based Institute of Nutrition and Food Safety found that more than 29% of children under 5 years old in China's poorest regions were growing at a slower than normal rate. This is quite different from the cities where too rich a diet has increased the level of obesity. In China's larger, wealthier cities milk, formula milk powder, yogurt, and many other types of food are available which would prevent childhood malnutrition. Yet, of course, the availability of such foods seems also to be viewed as a potential cause for the new Chinese "obesity epidemic." According to Chinese public health sources, severe obesity now affects some 16% to 20% of urban youngsters.[63] But, of course, "urban" itself is a highly problematic category, for it includes the rural Diaspora, living marginal lives in the large cities, as well as cities which have had little share in the new boom economy.

Now, in a China with a growing urban middle class, obesity seems to have been uncoupled from the official demand under Mao Zedong in 1979 that only one child per couple be allowed, which radically reduced the average of three or four children per family in rural areas and two or three in urban areas. China, unlike most societies in transformation that have a reduction in birth rate as a reflex of increasing economic status, saw the reduction in the number of children per family prior to the development of the new economic modernization begun under Deng Xiaoping. More food and more TV are today indeed a means of pampering these children, often called the "Little Emperors" (*xiao huangdi*)—but the number of children and their status are independent of economic change. These "Little Emperors" are "used to getting plenty of candy, lavish praise from grown-ups, and pretty much anything else [they] want."[64] And what they want is food, at least as imagined from the perspective of a Western observer writing for a Western audience accustomed to critiques of the "Fast Food Nation." They are imagined as being "weaned on cheeseburgers from McDonald's, pizza from Pizza Hut, and fried chicken from KFC." Their growing obesity has become not only a public health problem but a source for a new "weight-loss business." "At the Aimin Fat Reduction Hospital in Tianjin, a former military institution that launched China's first weight clinic in 1992, doctors treat 200 patients, most of them under 25, with a daily regimen of acupuncture, exercise, and healthy food.

Fifteen-year-old Liang Chen reports proudly that he has lost 33 lb. in less than a month at Aimin. But he can't stop reminiscing wistfully about his regular visits to KFC. (His favorite T-shirt is a souvenir from China's largest KFC store.) 'I used to be able to eat an entire family-size bucket all by myself,' he recalls. 'Just one?' snorts his roommate, 14-year-old Li Xiang. 'That's nothing. I used to be able to eat four buckets— sometimes five, if I didn't eat the corncobs and bread.' "[65]

Childhood obesity is not the only curse of the "Little Emperors," as anorexia nervosa seems also to be present. In 1993, an eating disorders clinic in the Fujien area reported 200 cases of radical underweight among children from 1988 to 1990. The balance between sexes was remarkable for anorexia nervosa from the Western point of view as 112 cases were boys and only 88 were girls. These cases were not the product of a starvation culture but rather of "non-fat phobic anorexia" caused, according to the researchers by the single-child policy as the children were spoiled by their parents and developed unhealthy eating habits, which contributed to their underweight.[66]

As the anthropologist Jun Jing notes from his fieldwork, things have changed radically since the 1980s. "Children now have more money and…their money goes to candy, cookies, chips, instant noodles, chocolate, nuts, soft drinks, and ice cream."[67] But even in his serious attempt to plumb the depths of the new obesity, the villain remains "Colonel Sanders, impeccable in his white suit and goatee, holding a jumbo bucket of Kentucky Fried Chicken."[68] Or at least Chicky (Qiqi) the Chinese cartoon emblem of KFC, the first Western food franchise in China (1987). This Chinese capitulation to Westernized (modern) food is paralleled by a sense of the nostalgia for a past of ideal foods, not specifically consumed by children. Thus, the essayist H. Y. Lowe (Wu Hsing-yuan) is quoted from 1939–40 (toward the end of the first epoch concerned with obesity) as expressing a nostalgia for the "eighteen kinds of foods and beverages that he had enjoyed as a child." As Jun Jing notes in his introduction only two ("dried cake powder" and "old rice powder") were specifically for children and "were intended to supplement mother's milk."[69] These were the "modern," manufactured foods advocated by the missionary physicians to augment the diet of hunger perceived in China.

Here the problem is not "Western" food but the absence of moderation, an absence fostered by the "Little Emperor" syndrome. The number of children is a result of the "old" Communist system and may be exacerbated by the availability of "Western" fast foods. Yet there are studies that minimize the shifts of diet in regard to a "Westernization" of the Chinese diet. One such study argues that while in the United States snacks contribute "more than one-third of their daily calories" and youths consume "a higher proportion of snack calories from foods prepared away from home" in "China...snacks provide only approximately 1% of energy. Fast food plays a much more dominant role in the American diet (approximately 20% of energy versus 2% to 7% in the other countries), but as yet does not contribute substantially to children's diets in the other countries. Urban–rural differences were found to be important, but narrowing over time, for China...whereas they are widening for Russia."[70] What has changed in contemporary China?

Moderation on the part of children is what has been sacrificed—not traditional foods. The status of the child may be linked to the new status of what the child eats, but childhood obesity is not the result of the availability of alternative, Western foods but the perceived special status of the child. No such parallel state existed in Japan where the reduction in the birthrate was concomitant with the increase of economic status. In Japan, American fast food has been omnipresent since the 1960s. If there is an increase of childhood obesity (and the argument is that this is then reflected in adult obesity) then it has occurred only over the past decade. In the National Survey of Primary and Middle Schools in Japan, between 1970 and 1997, obesity in 9-year-old children increased threefold but the focus has been on the past decade, a decade of economic retrenchment.[71]

Yet today in China no one would imagine tying childhood obesity to anything but perceived economic improvement in the "New Economy" as part of "Jiang Zemin's legacy." This, of course, mimics the Western *Super Size Me* rationale that sees all obesity as a result of the global "epidemic" of "junk food."[72] The Chinese term "kuaican" (actually "fast eating") does not have quite that pejorative sense, even though it contradicts the traditional notion that meals, at least, should be eaten slowly.[73] Yet a glance at the food diary of an 11-year-old boy written from June 7–14, 1997 reveals no Western "fast food" but a mix of "fast" but traditional noodle dishes and some candies and soft drinks.[74] This is much more in line with the traditional idea of "xiaochi" (small eats) that typified Chinese snack culture. Certainly not an "unhealthy" diet compared with the claims of the McDonaldization of teenage China.

The treatment for obesity also parallels the introduction of Westernized forms of "traditional" Chinese medicine. Thus "electroacupuncture" for the treatment of overweight has melded traditional views of obesity and the newest research on human metabolism, including serum total cholesterol, triglyceride, high-density lipoprotein cholesterol and low-density lipoprotein cholesterol.[75] What comes from the West can be cured now by that which (seems) indigenous to the East (but of course is not—just like obesity).

China, like America, is experiencing a new epidemic but one that documents its modernity—no model of Oriental, primitive infectious diseases here. Rather a claim of the "invasion from the West." However, the negative aspects of the new economy can be confronted through the importation of models of obesity from Western public health. Obesity and its treatment may both be understood as part of a system of modernization with all of the pitfalls recognized and the "cure" in sight.

VIII

GLOBESITY AND THE
PUBLIC'S HEALTH

The view that fat spreads across the map, spread by chickens or by genetic transmission across generations, means that there could be populations free from obesity. This fantasy of the Enlightenment physicians, of utopias where obesity could not exist because of the very nature of its inhabitants, their diet, their activities, reappears today with the public health model of globesity. The "French diet" and the "Chinese diet" as cures for obesity; the spread of McDonald's as the cause of obesity: all assume populations without even the potential for obesity. In 2001, the World Health Organization stated that there was a brand new pandemic of "globesity" sweeping the world. What is labeled as "globesity" is in fact the most recent iteration of an obsession with bodily control and the promise of universal health. Its modern iteration, however, comes with an unstated and complex history. If, said the ancients, you would only eat well, sacrifice to the gods, and avoid beans, then your health would improve or simply never decline. There have always been changes in eating patterns. Perhaps in the twenty-first century these changes speed around the world more quickly than in the past. But the notion of a world in decay due to the growth of girth carries with it odd and complex subtexts. What are the central implications of "globesity"?

"Globesity," according a publication of the Pan American Health Organization in 2002, "places the blame not on individuals but on globalization and development, with poverty as an exacerbating factor."[1] The focus on what have been called earlier in the twentieth century "diseases of extravagance" postulates a model not so much of change but of invasion—a Gresham's Law of Food in which the bad drives out the good. It is a modern version of "degeneracy theory," with the new assumption that the ills of the world are to be traced directly back to the developed world. In this way it is a dietary version of the basic global warming thesis: developed nations destroyed their environment and now they are invading the rest of the world, corrupting it. "Nature" was benign, even kind; now it has become threatening. "Globesity" argues that inherently healthy eating practices have been corrupted by the expansion of development and the resultant poverty. "Fat" is a product of globalization and modernity. The utopian "undeveloped" world, in Enlightenment jargon, the world of the "noble savage," is a world in which "diseases of extravagance" could not exist, as they are a reflex of a "civilized" model of exploitation and capitalism. The "cure" for "Globesity" in the twenty-first century is "natural" or "slow" food as a prophylactic against obesity as well as illness, as we have seen argued in the previous chapter. It is a return to the inherently "healthy" eating practices of the Edenic past.

Such views have a relatively long history. The French food writer, Jean Anthelme Brillat-Savarin, could write as late as 1825 that "Obesity is never found either among savages or in those classes of society, which must work in order to eat, or which do not eat except to exist." But he provided a caveat: "Savages will eat gluttonously and drink themselves insensible when ever they have a chance to."[2] This is very much in line with Immanuel Kant's view of "savages" and alcohol use in his lectures on anthropology first held in 1772–3 and published in 1798.[3] Obesity, therefore, could be an illness of natural man as well as of civilization because of the "savages'" weakness of will. Christoph Wilhelm Hufeland (1762–1836), who was, as we have seen earlier, one of the first modern medical commentators on dieting, recognized this when he commented that "a certain degree of cultivation is physically necessary for man, and promotes duration of life. The wild savage does not live so long as man in a state of civilization."[4]

The notion that the exotic can never be obese is one lodged in European tradition. Certainly humoral theory as adapted in the seventeenth century labeled exotics by their very nature as thin:

> Besides their scituation, hot and dry,
> Doth alwaies much obesity deny.
> Who ever saw a Spaniard over fat?
> Their Countrey-man (the SUN) prohibits that,
> Who by extensive heats exhals their moist,
> Unlesse perchance some Spaniard the Seas crost,
> And *Leiger* lay in *England* then he might
> Return a Shew, and the *Madrids* delight:[5]

"Fat" here is clearly the preferred state of being. The age of exploration extended the notion of a healthy and an unhealthy fat to the very bounds of the world to be documented by Enlightenment science.

This notion is also reflected in the memoirs of Georg Forster (1754–94) who accompanied Captain James Cook (1728–79) around the world in the 1770s. In 1773, Cook and Forster found themselves in Tahiti, an island that they saw as the perfect natural society. Food abounded, and one did not have to work for it. Therefore, gluttony was impossible, as only in a society of inadequacy did the passion for food arise. Fat men were impossible in Tahiti. Except, Forster reports that walking along the shore he saw a "very fat man, who seemed to be the chief of the district" being fed by a "woman who, sat near him, crammed down his throat by handfuls the remains of a large baked fish, and several breadfruits, which he swallowed with a voracious appetite." His face was the "picture of phlegmatic insensibility, and seemed to witness that all his thoughts centred in the care of his paunch." Forster is shocked because he had assumed that obesity of this nature was impossible in a world in which there was "a certain frugal equality in their way of living, and whose hours of enjoyment were justly proportioned to those of labour and rest." However, here was the proof that any society could have obese members, for in Tahiti Forster found a "luxurious individual spending his life in the most sluggish inactivity, and without one benefit to society, like the privileged parasites of more civilized climates, fattening on the superfluous produce of the soil, of which he robbed the labouring multitude."[6] This contradiction caused much consternation. Later Cook had recorded that in the language of the Society Isles the word for "obesity or corpulence" is *Oo'peea*.[7]

The belief in the inherent absence of obesity among "natural man" still echoes in Edwin James' 1819 statement that "The Missouri Indian is symmetrical and active, and in stature, equal, if not somewhat superior, to the ordinary European standard; tall men are numerous. The active occupations of war and hunting, together perhaps with the occasional privations to which they are subjected, prevents that unsightly obesity, so often a concomitant of civilization, indolence, and serenity of mental temperament."[8] But this is true only of men. John Wyeth observed in 1832 that among the tribes of the Northwest "The persons of the men generally are rather symmetrical; their stature is low, with light sinewy limbs, and remarkably small delicate hands. The women are usually more rotund, and, in some instances, even approach obesity."[9] Among "natural peoples" it is as shocking to imagine a fat man then as now.

The idea of where "natural man" is to be found is, of course, not limited to the exotic, only to the utopian. Thus, in an essay of the difference between the Scots and the English published in 1819 the former are described as "a race of tall, well-formed people, active of limb and powerful of muscle; leaner by far than the English (for here a very fat man is stared at, and one of such bulk as is met with at every corner in London, must, it would seem, lay his account with a little quizzing from all his friends on the subject of his obesity.)"[10] This is an image from the age of Sir Walter Scott's Waverley novels and his positive revitalization of a Scots identity in the Regency period. The Scot is "natural man" in comparison to the obese, short, inactive Englishman. This is a caricature often applied to the Prince Regent, the future George IV, by artists such as James Gillray in his image "A Voluptuary under the Horrors of Digestion" (July 2, 1792). Indeed the writer and critic Leigh Hunt spent 1813 and 1814 in prison for writing in 1812 (among other things) that the Prince Regent was a "fat Adonis of Fifty."[11] It is not good always to speak truth to power—if the power is truly obese.

The negative counterpart to "natural man" in the thought of the time was the scholar. Thus there are regimens of dieting for

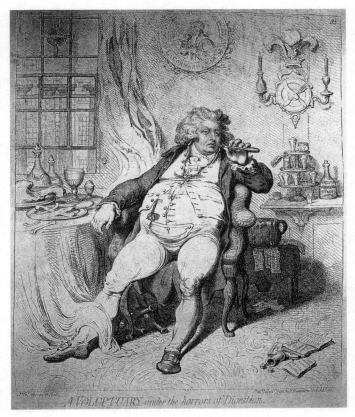

17. James Gillray, "A Voluptary under the Horrors of Digestion." (1792) (*Wellcome Collection*)

intellectuals. In 1825, the American Chandler Robbins suggested that the "evils usually incident to sedentary and studious habits" were the result of poor diet.[12] Yet the author also noted that what was an appropriate diet for one did not always work for others.[13] The key was variety, temperature

163

(cool was better than hot, such as food eaten in nature), frequency (three meals a day, one "liberal" and two "slight"), the avoidance of exercise (after a meal one should rest) and "chewing long and leisurely": "masticate, denticate, chump, grind, and swallow." This later becomes gospel by the end of the nineteenth century, as espoused by Horace Fletcher, but it is, in the end, one thing that "maintains vigour of the mind and the body, temperance becomes the parent of all other virtues," unlike what reportedly happens in the idyllic world of "natural man."[14] In 1836, William Newnham observed in London that "overstimulation of the brain" caused "the general health to suffer."[15] What results is torpor, and the cure is dieting. Mastication is vital but the diet must be "simple: animal food under dressed, roast in preference to boil'd; let vegetables be very much dressed, and bread very much baked; sauces, made dishes, and pastry to be avoided, or taken very sparingly."[16] Water should be taken, rather than wine. Indeed, the cure for the scholar is the diet of "natural man."

There had been a debate about whether those natives labeled as "degenerate" also suffered from obesity. As I have argued elsewhere, the classic example of the degenerate native was found in the Khoi-Khoi (Hottentots) of Southern Africa, who through the eighteenth century and beyond were labeled as huge and deformed.[17] Francis Galton made his reputation as one of the first "scientist-explorers" in South Africa in 1852. His account of that trip catapulted him to fame as a geographer. He was impressed by the girth of the inhabitants. When he meets Nagoro, the king of the Ovampo, according to one of his informants "the fattest man in the world and, larger than either of my wagons,"[18] he is struck initially by "an amazingly fat old fellow...he was very short of breath, and...waddled up looking very severe…"[19] He is indeed "obese,"[20] But he is not the only one:

> Mr. Hahn's household was large. There was an interpreter, and a sub-interpreter, and again others; but all most excellently well-behaved, and showing to great advantage the influence of their master. These servants were chiefly Hottentots, who had migrated with Mr. Hahn from Hottentot-land, and, like him, had picked up the language of the Damaras. The sub-interpreter was married to a charming person, not only a Hottentot in figure, but in that respect a Venus among Hottentots. I was perfectly aghast at her development, and made inquiries upon that delicate point as far as I dared among my missionary friends. The result is, that I believe Mrs. Petrus to be the lady who ranks second among all the Hottentots for the beautiful outline that her back affords, Jonker's wife ranking as the first; the latter, however, was slightly passée, while Mrs. Petrus was in full *embonpoint*. I profess to be a scientific man, and was exceedingly anxious to obtain accurate measurements of her shape; but there was great difficulty in doing this. I did not know a word of Hottentot, and could never therefore have explained to the lady what the object of my foot rule could be; and I really dared not ask my worthy missionary host to interpret for me. I therefore felt in a dilemma as I gazed at her form, that gift of bounteous nature to this favoured race, which no mantua-maker, with all her crinoline and stuffing, can do otherwise but humbly imitate. The object of my admiration stood under a tree, and was turning herself about to all points of the compass, as ladies who wish to be admired usually do. Of a sudden my eye fell upon my sextant; the bright thought struck me, and I took a series of observations upon her figure in every direction, up and down, crossways, diagonally, and so forth, and I registered them carefully upon an outline drawing for fear of any mistake; this being done, I boldly pulled out my measuring

tape, and having thus obtained both base and angles, I worked out the results by trigonometry and logarithms.[21]

Yet there were counter voices who earlier saw in the Hottentots the "noble savage" and this quality was measured by their lack of girth: "The Hottentots are neither so small of stature nor so deformed as some have described them...Both sexes...are well made; keeping a due medium between leanness and obesity."[22] Were the Africans unduly large or were they healthily "normal"? This was answered with the development of "tropical medicine."

Allopathic medicine "discovers" the evolving spread of diseases of civilization to the world of natural man as an offshoot of colonial medicine. The standard handbooks of what comes to be called "tropical" medicine are little concerned with the diseases of the West in the rest of the world.[23] Michael Gelfand, in his *The Sick African* (1944) is still concerned only with the differential diagnosis of diseases of Westerners in Africa and of the "natives." He is much more focused on the diseases that Westerners can get in Africa, than those diseases of encroaching "civilization" suffered by Africans. Thus the only discussions of nutritional diseases are those of vitamin deficiency (such as pellagra), and the only discussion of obesity is as a specific problem of the failure of the pituitary gland.[24]

Yet there were other voices to be heard. Cyril Percy Donnison argued in 1937 that "civilization" was the cause of disease; indeed was itself a harbinger of diseases.[25] Cultures, for Donnison, follow a series of developmental changes in terms of their psychological and social constitution. He had worked as a medical officer in Kenya, with "a primitive native race in a fairly isolated part of Africa"[26] and was surprised at the lack of

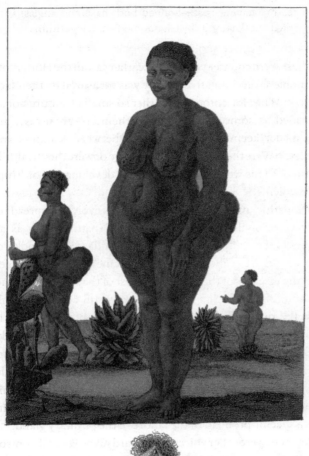

18. A female Hottentot, possibly Saartjie 'Sarah' Baartman, with a disease (steatopygy), which results in a protuberance of the buttocks due to an abnormal accumulation of fat. From *Journal Complémentaire du Dictionaire Des Sciences Médicales* (Paris: C. L. F. Panckoucke, 1819). (*Wellcome Collection*)

167

"Western" diseases, such as "high blood pressure, diabetes, exophthalmic goiter, peptic ulcer," which he attributed to the absence of Western civilization. For him, Western civilization, marked by rapid change, was inherently different from the "'primitive' races," where the "same conditions persist for a large number of generations." But by the 1930s he saw "the spread of the diseases of the white races to other parts of the world to which White civilization has spread,"[27] into "primitive" societies as well as into "Ancient" civilizations such as China.[28] Among these were "diseases of nutrition."[29] He contrasted the inherent diseases of starvation with those "conditions due to overnutrition":

> Adiposity is rare in the primitive native but is seen occasionally in mild degree in towns and is common in the American Negro...Overnutrition seems to be associated with the civilized state.[30]

The reason given is the "lessened expenditure of physical energy and increased accessibility to food supply."[31] Julian Huxley made a similar remark in 1930 on a trip to Africa when he observed that "almost the only fat woman I saw in Africa worked in a Nairobi brewery" and mused that beer might be fattening.[32] The evolution of "Western diseases" and the concomitant praise of "natural man" becomes the mantra that underlies "globesity." As late as 1981 Hugh Trowell, looking back to the 1920s and his service in colonial Africa, commented that, "In 1926 when I started medical work in Kenya obesity was rare. At the present the towns of east Africa contain many fat upper class Africans, who are grossly obese." The cause is the "change of energy foods" and the introduction of "fibre free fat and sugar."[33]

Donnison condemns what seems to underlie many of the discourses about "globesity." He puts both the dieting culture and the food faddist in the camp of those who misconstrue the nature of causation of "Western diseases":

> The food faddist never finds difficulty in adapting the facts to determine the root of all evil to lie in his particular aversion, whatever that might be, whilst the newer methods of preserving, distributing, and preparing food stuffs present, superficially, a tempting target for attack. Others see deficient or ill-balanced diet as responsible for nearly all our ills—the criteria of balance always being obscure.[34]

He notes that civilization provides access to food that "primitive" societies cannot have: "Few native races have such abundant access to food that consistent overnutrition is practicable."[35] In Western civilization, more food is available because of improved transportation and agricultural methods; food is more elaborately prepared; and is also more attractively presented.[36] But he does not fault overnutrition "in large measure" for the pathologies he associates with civilization as he believes that one should not condemn modern dietetic practices for their negative impact. The "'primitive' races" are more often ill because of the "unhygienic feeding" now eliminated in civilization.

In 1939, a Cleveland dentist named Weston Price (1870–1948) self-published *Nutrition and Physical Degeneration*, which argued that isolated cultures showed no tooth decay and less arthritis, diabetes, cancer and heart disease than people living in urbanized, industrialized nations.[37] This seemed to make some sense at the time given the politics of food faddism, except that Price, as with all of the earliest advocates of "natural man," also sees such societies as better, purer, and more moral than more developed societies, which show "character changes" and are in a state of "moral deterioration."[38] The communities, including dairy farmers in Switzerland's Loetschental Valley, the Aborigines of Australia, the "Gaelics" in the Outer and Inner Hebrides, Maoris in New Zealand and native peoples in ancient and modern Peru, as well as the Melanesians and Polynesians (remember Forster) were so varied and had such radically different food cultures that Price focused on the absence of processed foods, such as refined sugar and flour, and hydrogenated oils. His goal is a "nutritional program for race regeneration." Contemporary society has deficient foods for the Western urban dweller, which is the source of inadequate nutrition among the "native."

The result of colonial expansion is the encroachment of corrupt civilization on the healthy, natural world.[39] For Price, (and his views on nutrition at least have lasted) "natural man" is healthy because natural man eats "natural" foods, a claim belied by the complex reality of such cultures, as observers in the eighteenth century could well have shown him. Indeed, his example comes from "the high Alps of Switzerland," where he found "an excellent state of physical development and health in adults and children living in the high valleys." This state of health persists in spite of the inroads of "refined cereals, a high intake of sweets, canned goods, sweetened fruits, chocolate; and a greatly reduced use of dairy products" among the urban Swiss.[40] His explanation for the innate "healthiness" of those Swiss "isolated" from the spread of modern, manufactured and, therefore, corrupting foods is the consumption of "rye...the only cereal that developed well for human food."[41] He took a piece of the rye bread and had it analysed, finding that "it was rich in minerals and vitamins."

A hundred years before, he would have found the valleys full of "cretins" with the stigmata of degeneration, the goiter, clearly present, as B. A. Morel (1809–73), who based his work on "degeneration" on these cases in 1857, saw it. All would be suffering from severe mental retardation—caused by the absence of iodine. Or they would have been simply "mad" from eating rye grain covered with ergot, a poisonous fungus. Swiss public health officials intervened over the subsequent fifty years; they turned the verdant valleys of the Alps into Price's Edenic landscape, where only healthy food is consumed. Even "natural man" needs civilization.

Today, we are attempting to reverse the argument. Eat organically, eat naturally, eat healthily, eat fat-free, eat high-fiber, eat low-carb, eat slowly (or, at least, eat slow food), and you are by definition a better person than those who don't. Companies such as "Whole Foods" juxtapose "conventional" and "organic" foods much to the advantage of the "organic," which seems closer to nature. "Slow" food is more natural than "fast" food. Ironically the boom in the sale of kosher food (which only means ritually supervised) in the United States today has much the same health rationale. As one American hot dog maker's advertizement has it—kosher food answers to a higher authority—but it also carries with it the promise of more natural eating. Eat like our Paleolithic ancestors, say the advocates of the *Paleolithic Prescription*, and you will be healthier and more morally attuned to the world.[42] It is the claim of the return to the natural that is seen as the answer to "globesity." Almost everything offers that promise now. But only as long as the strict guidelines of civilization as to health, cleanliness, adequate labeling, workers' rights, and fairly traded foods are not compromised (something I am sure that Paleolithic peoples could not have imagined during their extremely short, brutal, and disease-plagued lives). Maybe, at the end of the day, our desire to control and reform our bodies is what is truly "modern" and the obesity epidemic is only proof of our desire to undertake this quixotic task.

GLOSSARY

ALLOPATHIC according to the World Health Association in 2001 the broad category of medical practice that is sometimes called scientific medicine or biomedicine.

ANOREXIA NERVOSA self-imposed starvation, which came to be a psychiatric syndrome clearly delineated by physical signs and symptoms and which was understood to have a psychogenic origin. The name, anorexia nervosa, was coined by William Gull in 1868. In the 1920s, the view of Morris Simmonds dominated: anorexia was the result of a lesion of the pituitary gland. It was only after World War II that Hilde Bruch began to speak of the lack of self-esteem and a distorted body image caused by maternal rejection in such patients.

BARIATRIC SURGERY the practice of bypassing parts of the digestive tract to allow a morbidly obese patient (body mass index greater than 40) to lose weight either through consuming less food or through malabsorption. Malabsorption refers to food passing directly through the digestive tract without the nutrients being absorbed by the body. This practice is only recommended for patients for whom other weight loss options, including medical diets, have failed.

BODY MASS INDEX (BMI) a mathematical value calculated by weight in kilograms divided by height in meters squared

(kg/m^2). It remains the prime indicator for the definition of obesity today and is highly correlated with health risk. Thus, today underweight is indicated by a BMI of less than 18.5; normal weight by a BMA of 18.5 to 24.9; overweight by a BMI of 25 to 29.9; and obesity by a BMI of 30 or greater.

CALORIE a scientific unit of measurement that describes the amount of energy contained in a substance. As a term it has had a wide range of meanings. Coined in France in the 1830s, it was adopted into English in the 1870s.

DIETING has in the twenty-first century come to mean the control of the intake of nutrients and the use of parallel interventions, such as exercise, psychological therapy, surgery, or pharmaceuticals to control (increase or decrease) body weight, strength, health, or shape.

ETIOLOGY the causes of a disease or the method by which a disease is constructed.

GENETICS the science of heredity and variation in living organisms. The modern science of genetics, which seeks to understand the process of inheritance, only began with the work of Gregor Mendel in the mid-nineteenth century.

GLOBALIZATION an ongoing process by which regional economies, societies, and cultures have become integrated through a globe-spanning network of communication and exchange.

GLOBESITY (global obesity), a term coined in 2001 by the World Health Organization to label the worldwide epidemic of obesity.

HORMONE a signaling compound or molecule in the body that enables one part of the body to communicate with another

part of the body. The term appears first in the scientific literature in the opening decade of the twentieth century.

HUMORS the *chymoi*. The four crucial bodily fluids in classical
Greek medicine, blood, yellow bile, black bile, and phlegm,
which were found in all individuals, and produced health
when in balance and illness when one dominated over the
others.

ILEUM the last portion of the small intestine.

INFECTION a detrimental colonization of a host organism by
a foreign species. In an infection, the infecting organism
seeks to utilize the host's resources to multiply, usually at
the expense of the host.

INFECTOBESITY infectious obesity, a term coined by Nikhil
Dhurandhar and Richard Atkinson, when they argued that
obesity could be caused in part by an infectious agent,
adenovirus-36 (Ad-36).

JEJUNUM the middle part of the small intestine.

JEJUNOILEAL BYPASS a surgical intervention, where the
beginning of the jejunum is connected to the end of the
ileum.

MATERIALISM a philosophic position that holds that the
only thing that exists is matter; that all things are composed
of material and all phenomena are the result of material
interactions.

MORAL PANIC an "episode, condition, person, or group of
persons" that have in recent times, been "defined as a threat
to societal values and interests." (Stanley Cohen) Coined by
Jock Young in his 1971 study of the beginnings of the
British drug scene.

NEURASTHENIA a syndrome of chronic mental and physical weakness and fatigue, which was thought to be caused by exhaustion of the nervous system.

OBESITY is not itself a "disease" but rather a phenomenological category that reflects the visible manifestation of body size, which potentially can have multiple (as well as multifactorial) causes.

PTOMAINE a form of toxin, formed by decarboxylation of an amino acid, perhaps by bacteria.

SOMATIC of the body, rather than the mind.

VEGETARIANISM the practice of following a diet based on plant-based foods. Thomas Tyron (1634–1703), in his *The Way to Wealth, Long Life and Happiness*, first and most dramatically linked vegetarianism to the original ways of Eve and Adam in Gen. 1: 29. Man could return to paradise, but only if he ate no meat.

NOTES

Prologue

1. Jock Young, "The Role of the Police as Amplifiers of Deviance; Negotiators of Drug Control as Seen in Notting Hill," in Stanley Cohen, ed., *Images of Deviance* (Harmondsworth, England: Penguin, 1971), 27–61.

2. Donna Eberwine, "Globesity: The Crisis of Growing Proportions," *Perspectives in Health*, 7 (3) (2002), 6–11; here, 8.

Chapter 1

1. David T.-D. Clarke, *Daniel Lambert*, Leicestershire Museums Publication 23 (1981), 3.

2. Jan Bondeson, *The Two-headed Boy and Other Medical Marvels* (Ithaca, NY: Cornell University Press, 2000), 243.

3. T. Coe, "A Letter… Concerning Mr. Bright, the Fat Man at Malden in Essex," *The Royal Society: Philosophical Transactions*, 47 (1751–2), 188–9.

4. Coe, "Concerning Mr. Bright," 189.

5. Coe, "Concerning Mr. Bright," 191.

6. Coe, "Concerning Mr. Bright," 192.

7. William Harvey, *On Corpulence in Relation to Disease: With Some Remarks on Diet* (London: Henry Renshaw, 1872), viii.

8. Charles Dickens, *The Pickwick Papers*, ed. James Kinsley (Oxford: Clarendon Press, 1986), 61.

9. Dickens, *Pickwick Papers*, 340.

10. Dickens, *Pickwick Papers*, 344.

11. Dickens, *Pickwick Papers*, 675.

12. Dickens, *Pickwick Papers*, 94.

13. Dickens, *Pickwick Papers*, 94.

14. Dickens, *Pickwick Papers*, 89.

15. Wilhelm Ebstein, *Die Fettleibigkeit (Corpulenz) und ihre Behand-lung nach physiologischen Grundsätzen*, 6th edn. (Wiesbaden: J. F. Bergmann, 1884). Cited from *Corpulence and Its Treatment on Physiological Principles*, trans. A. H. Keane (London: H. Grevel, 1884), 11.

16. Dickens, *Pickwick Papers*, 685–6.

17. Dickens, *Pickwick Papers*, 686.

18. Dickens, *Pickwick Papers*, 712–3.

19. W. G. Don, "Remarkable Case of Obesity in a Hindoo Boy aged Twelve Years," *The Lancet*, 73 (April 9, 1859), 363.

20. Edward Jukes, *On Indigestion and Costiveness; a Series of Hints To Both Sexes...* (London: John Churchill, 1833), 287.

21. Jukes, *On Indigestion and Costiveness*, 289–90.

22. "A Case of Narcolepsy," *The Lancet*, 142 (July 8, 1893), 100.

23. "The Fat Boy of Peckham," *The Lancet*, 163 (January 9, 1904), 106.

24. William Ord, "The Bradshaw Lecture on Myxoedema and Allied Disorders," *The Lancet*, 152 (November 12, 1898), 1243–8; here, 1246.

25. Ord, "The Bradshaw Lecture," 1246.

26. E. Watson-Williams, "Obesity," *The Lancet*, 143 (August 15, 1953), 343.

27. H. Letheby Tidy, "An Address on Dyspituitarism, Obesity, and Infantilism," *The Lancet*, 203 (September 16, 1922): 567–602; references here on 600.

28. Tidy, "An Address on Dyspituitarism, Obesity, and Infantilism," 600.

29. M. H. Kryger, "Fat, Sleep and Charles Dickens: Literary and Medical Contributions to the Understanding of Sleep Apnea," *Clinics in Chest Medicine*, 6 (1985), 555–62; K. Tjoorstad, "Pickwick-syndromet. Fra litteraere spekulasjoner til sovnforskning," *Tidsskr Nor Laegeforen*, 115 (1995), 3,768–72; Uwe Henrik Peters, *Das Pickwick-Syndrom: Schlafänfalle und Periodenatmung bei Adiposen* (München: Urban und Schwarzenberg, 1976).

30. C. Sidney Burwell, Eugene D. Robin, Robert D. Whaley, and Albert G. Bickelman, "Extreme Obesity Associated with Alveolar Hypoventilation—A Pickwickian Syndrome," *American Journal of Medicine*, 21 (1956), 811–18; see also Antoine Cuvelier and Jean-François Muir, "Obesity-hypoventilation Syndrome and Noninvasive Mechanical Ventilation: New Insights in the *Pickwick Papers?*" *Chest*, 131 (2007), 7–8 and Karen Spruyt and David Gozal, "Mr. Pickwick and His Child Went on a Field Trip and Returned Almost Empty Handed… What We Do Not Know and Imperatively Need to Learn About Obesity and Breathing During Sleep in Children!" *Sleep Medicine Reviews*, 12 (2008), 335–8.

31. P. Potvliege, "Le syndrome 'de Pickwick.' Priorité de sa description par le duc de Saint-Simon (1675–1755)," *Nouvelle Presse Médicale*, 11 (1982), 2360.

32. As have subsequent studies: see John G. Sotos, "Taft and Pickwick: Sleep Apnea in the White House," *Chest*, 124 (2003), 1133–42.

33. N. Spier and S. Karelitz, "The Pickwickian Syndrome: A Case in a Child," *American Journal of Diseases of Childhood*, 99 (1960), 822–7; G. G. Cayler, J. Mays, and H. D. Riley, Jr., "Cardiorespiratory Syndrome of Obesity (Pickwickian Syndrome) in Children," *Pediatrics*, 27 (1961), 237–45.

34. Dickens, *Pickwick Papers*, 48.

35. Hilde Bruch, *Eating Disorders: Obesity, Anorexia Nervosa, and the Person Within* (London: Routledge and Kegan Paul, 1974), p. 137.

36. S. P. Kalra, M. Bagnasco, E. E. Otukonyong, M. G. Dube, and P. S. Kalra, "Rhythmic, Reciprocal Ghrelin and Leptin Signaling:

New Insight in the Development of Obesity," *Regulatory Peptides*, 111 (2003), 1–11.

37. Claudio Rabec, "Leptin, Obesity and Control of Breathing: The New Adventures of Mr. Pickwick," *Revista Electrónica de Biomedicina / Electronic Journal of Biomedicine*, 1 (2006), 3–7.

38. A. A. Conti, A. Conti, and G. F. Gensini, "Fat Snorers and Sleepy-Heads: Were Many Distinguished Characters of the Past Affected by the Obstructive Sleep Apnea Syndrome?" *Medical Hypothesis*, 67 (4) (2006), 975–9.

39. E. Bilavsky, H. Yarden-Bilavsky, and S. Ashkenazi, "Literature Names for Pediatric Medical Conditions," *Acta Paediatrica*, 96 (2007), 975–8.

40. Cited by James Mackenzie, *The History of Health and the Art of Preserving It* (Edinburgh: William Gordon, 1758), 121.

Chapter 2

1. Hippocrates, "Aphorisms," in *Hippocrates, Volume IV. Nature of Man. Regimen in Health. Humours. Aphorisms. Regimen 1–3. Dreams. Heracleitus. On the Universe*, trans. W. H. S. Jones (Cambridge, MA: Harvard University Press, 1931); (*Aphorisms* V, XLVI).

2. Hippocrates, "Aphorisms," (*Aphorisms* II, XLIV).

3. Hippocrates, "Aphorisms," (*Aphorisms* I, IV).

4. Aristotle, "On Length and Shortness of Life," in *Aristotle, Volume VIII. On the Soul. Parva Naturalia. On Breath*, trans. W. S. Hett (Cambridge, MA: Harvard University Press, 1936), 403.

5. Aristotle, "On Length and Shortness of Life," 403.

6. Aristotle, "On Length and Shortness of Life," 407.

7. Hippocrates, "Aphorisms," (*Aphorisms* I, III).

8. Celsus, *De medicina*, trans. W. G. Spencer (Cambridge, MA: Harvard University Press, 1935), vol. I, 97.

9. Galen, *Galen on the Properties of Foodstuffs*, trans. Owen Powell (Cambridge: Cambridge University Press, 2003), 45.

10. Paulus Aegineta, *The Seven Books of Paulus Aegineta*, 3 vols., trans. Francis Adams (London: Sydenham Society, 1844), vol. I, 81.

11. Paulus Aegineta, *The Seven Books*, vol. I, 81.

12. Lev. 11:3; Deut. 14:6.

13. Lev. 11:9; Deut. 14:9.

14. Deut. 12:21.

15. Judg. 3: 17, 22.

16. Augustine, *Confessions*, trans. R. S. Pine-Coffin (London: Penguin Books, 1961), 235–7.

17. I Cor. 8:8.

18. Augustine, *The City of God*. 7 vols. (Cambridge: Harvard University Press, 1957–72), II: 247 and III: 37.

19 1 Cor. 8.1.

20. W. F. Toal, ed., *The Sunday Sermons of the Great Fathers*, 4 vols., (Chicago: Regnery, 1957–63), 3: 315.

21. Saint Teresa of Avila, *The Life of Saint Teresa of Avila By Herself* (Harmondsworth: Penguin, 1957).

22. P. Holland, trans. *Regimen sanitatis salernitanum*. Reprinted in John Sinclair, ed., *The Code of Health and Longevity*, 4 vols. (Edinburgh: Arch. Constable & Co., 1806), III: 5–46; here, 35.

23. P. Holland, *Regimen sanitatis salernitanum*, 7.

24. P. Holland, *Regimen sanitatis salernitanum*, 19.

Chapter 3

1. Luigi Cornaro, *The Art of Living Long* (Milwaukee: William F. Butler, 1903), 41.

2. Luigi Cornaro, *The Art of Living Long*, 42.

3. Luigi Cornaro, *The Art of Living Long*, 43–4.

4. Luigi Cornaro, *The Art of Living Long*, 44.

5. Luigi Cornaro, *The Art of Living Long*, 40.

6. Luigi Cornaro, *The Art of Living Long*, 41.

7. Luigi Cornaro, *The Art of Living Long*, 42.

8. Luigi Cornaro, *The Art of Living Long*, 46.

9. Luigi Cornaro, *The Art of Living Long*, 87–8.

10. Luigi Cornaro, *The Art of Living Long*, 48.

11. Luigi Cornaro, *The Art of Living Long*, 69–70.

12. Sanctorius Sanctorius, *De statica medicina*. Reprinted in *The Code of Health*, John Sinclair, ed., *The Code of Health and Longevity*, 4 vols. (Edinburgh: Arch. Constable & Co., 1806), III, 122–230; here, 129.

13. La Bruyère, *Characters*, trans. Jean Stewart (Baltimore: Penguin, 1970), 208.

14. Giovanni Baptista Morgagni, *Epistola anatomica clinical XXI: de sedibus et Causis Morborum per anatomen indagata* (Patavii: Sumptibus Remondinianis, 1765).

15. Christopher William Hufeland, *The Art of Prolonging Life* (London: J. Bell, 1797), 1: 169.

16. Hufeland, *The Art of Prolonging Life*, 2: 43.

17. Hufeland, *The Art of Prolonging Life*, 2: 43.

18. Hufeland, *The Art of Prolonging Life*, 2: 45–6.

19. Hufeland, *The Art of Prolonging Life*, 2: 242.

20. Hufeland, *The Art of Prolonging Life*, 2: 248.

21. Hufeland, *The Art of Prolonging Life*, 2: 64.

22. Hufeland, *The Art of Prolonging Life*, 2: 217.

23. Hufeland, *The Art of Prolonging Life*, 2: 9.

24. Immanuel Kant, "Von der Macht des Gemüts, durch den blossen Vorsatz seiner krankhaften Gefühle Meister zu sein," in Wilhelm Weischedel, ed., *Immanuel Kant, Schriften zur*

Anthropologie, Geschichtsphilosophie, Politik und Pädagogik, I (*Werkausgabe*, vol. XI) (Frankfurt: Suhrkamp, 1991), 371–93.

25. Kant, "Von der Macht des Gemüts," 375.

26. Kant, "Von der Macht des Gemüts," 383.

27. Paul M. Zall, *Ben Franklin's Humor* (Lexington, Kentucky: The University Press of Kentucky, 2005), 163.

28. Gilbert Chinard, ed., *Benjamin Franklin on The Art of Eating: Together with the Rules of Health and Long Life and the Rules to Find Out a Fit Measure of Meat and Drink, with Several Recipes* (Princeton: Princeton University Press, 1958), 12.

29. Thomas Jameson, *Essays on the Changes of the Human Body, at its Different Ages* (London: Longman, Hurst, Rees, Orme, and Brown, 1811).

30. Jameson, *Essays on the Changes of the Human Body*, 90.

31. Jameson, *Essays on the Changes of the Human Body*, 91.

32. Jameson, *Essays on the Changes of the Human Body*, 91.

33. Jameson, *Essays on the Changes of the Human Body*, 92.

34. Jameson, *Essays on the Changes of the Human Body*, 105.

35. George Cheyne, *The English Malady; or, A Treatise of Nervous Diseases of All Kinds, as Spleen, Vapours, Lowness of Spirits, Hypochondriacal and Hysterical Distempers* (London: Strahan in Cornhill, 1733), 325.

36. Cheyne, *The English Malady*, 325.

37. Cheyne, *The English Malady*, 326.

38. Cheyne, *The English Malady*, 328.

39. Cheyne, *The English Malady*, 331.

40. Cheyne, *The English Malady*, 334.

41. Cheyne, *The English Malady*, 337.

42. Cheyne, *The English Malady*, 338.

43. Cheyne, *The English Malady*, 342.

44. Cheyne, *The English Malady*, 342.

45. Cheyne, *The English Malady*, 346.

46. Cheyne, *The English Malady*, 348.

47. Cheyne, *The English Malady*, 350.

48. Cheyne, *The English Malady*, 353.

49. Cheyne, *The English Malady*, 355.

50. Cheyne, *The English Malady*, 358.

51. Cheyne, *The English Malady*, 361.

52. John Wesley, *Primitive Physic: or, An Easy and Natural Method of Curing Most Diseases*. 14th edn. (Bristol: William Pine, 1770), xvii.

53. Wesley, *Primitive Physic*, xviii.

54. Wesley, *Primitive Physic*, 43.

Chapter 4

1. Thomas Reid, *The Works of Thomas Reid*, ed. William Hamilton (Edinburgh: Maclachan and Stewart, 1854), 235.

2. Jean Anthelme Brillat-Savarin, *The Physiology of Taste: Or Meditations on Transcendental Gastronomy*, trans. M. F. K. Fisher (Washington: Counterpoint, 1999), 245.

3. Samuel Johnson, *Diaries, Prayers, and Annals*, in E. L. McAdam, Jr., D. Hyde, and M. Hyde, eds., *The Yale Edition of the Works of Samuel Johnson* (New Haven: Yale University Press, 1958), I: 301.

4. James Boswell, *Life of Johnson*, ed. R. W. Chapman (Oxford: Oxford University Press, 1980), 958.

5. Boswell, *Life of Johnson*, 958.

6. Boswell, *Life of Johnson*, 958.

7. Boswell, *Life of Johnson*, 1121.

8. William Banting, *Letter on Corpulence, Addressed to the Public*. 3rd edn. (London: Harrison, 1864), 10–1.

9. Banting, *Letter on Corpulence*, 13.

10. Banting, *Letter on Corpulence*, 15.

11. Banting, *Letter on Corpulence*, 16.

12. Banting, *Letter on Corpulence*, 14.

13. Banting, *Letter on Corpulence*, 14.

14. Banting, *Letter on Corpulence*, 28.

15. Banting, *Letter on Corpulence*, 14.

16. Banting, *Letter on Corpulence*, 13.

17. Banting, *Letter on Corpulence*, 20.

18. William Harvey, *On Corpulence in Relation to Disease: With Some Remarks on Diet* (London: Henry Renshaw, 1872), 69.

19. Harvey, *On Corpulence in Relation to Disease*, 17.

20. Brillat-Savarin, *The Physiology of Taste*, 196.

21. Brillat-Savarin, *The Physiology of Taste*, 197.

22. Banting, *Letter on Corpulence*, 22–3.

23. Banting, *Letter on Corpulence*, 21.

24. A. W. Moore, *Corpulency, i.e., Fat, or Embonpoint, in Excess* (London: Frederick William Ruston, 1857).

25. Watson Bradshaw, *On Corpulence* (London: Philip & Son, 1864).

26. Bradshaw, *On Corpulence*, 6.

27. "A London Physician," *How to Get Fat or the Means of Preserving the Medium Between Leanness and Obesity* (London: John Smith, 1865).

28. "A London Physician," *How to Get Fat*, 7.

29. Harvey, *On Corpulence in Relation to Disease*, vi.

30. Harvey, *On Corpulence in Relation to Disease*, ix.

31. William E. Aytoun, "Banting on Corpulence," *Blackwood's Edinburgh Magazine*, 96 (November 1864), 607–17.

32. Ellen G. White, *Early Writings* [1882] (Hagerstown, MD: Review and Herald Publishing House, 2000), 184.

33. White, *Early Writings*, 184.

34. J. H. Kellogg, *The Stomach: Its Disorders, and How to Cure Them* (London: International Tract Society, 1896), 17.

35. Kellogg, *The Stomach*, 19.

36. Kellogg, *The Stomach*, 55.

37. Kellogg, *The Stomach*, 58.

38. Kellogg, *The Stomach*, 112.

39. Kellogg, *The Stomach*, 105.

40. Kellogg, *The Stomach*, 96.

41. Kellogg, *The Stomach*, 227 ff.

42. J. H. Kellogg, *The Home Book of Modern Medicine* (London: C. D. Cazenove & Sons, 1907), 593.

43. Kellogg, *The Home Book of Modern Medicine*, 1561.

44. Catharine Beecher, *Miss Beecher's Domestic Receipt Book Designed as a Supplement to the Treatise on Domestic Economy.* (New York: Harper, 1846).

45. 1 Pet. 2:11.

46. Sylvester Graham, *Lecture to Young Men on Chastity.* 2nd edn. (Boston: Light & Stearns, 1837), 29.

47. Graham, *Lecture to Young Men on Chastity*, 16.

48. Graham, *Lecture to Young Men on Chastity*, 40.

49. Graham, *Lecture to Young Men on Chastity*, 60.

50. Graham, *Lecture to Young Men on Chastity*, 92.

51. Sylvester Graham, *The Physiology of Feeding, Consisting of the Three Lectures on Diet from "The Science of Human Life"* (London: Ideal Publishing Union, 1897).

52. Graham, *The Physiology of Feeding*, 115.

53. Graham, *The Physiology of Feeding*, 150.

54. Henry Perky, *Wisdom vs. Foolishness* (Worcester: The Perky Publishing Co., 1902), 86.

55. Perky, *Wisdom vs. Foolishness*.

56. C. W. Post, *I am Well! The Modern Practice of Natural Suggestion as Distinct from Hypnotic Unnatural Influence* (Boston: Lee and Shepard, 1895), 4.

57. Peyton John Paxson, *Charles William Post: The Mass Marketing of Health and Welfare*, Dissertation (Boston University, 1993), 36.

58. Paxson, *Charles William Post*, 193.

59. Paxson, *Charles William Post*, 191.

60. Paxson, *Charles William Post*, 203.

61. Paxson, *Charles William Post*, 325.

62. R. Marie Griffith, *Born Again Bodies: Flesh and Spirit in American Christianity* (Berkeley: University of California Press, 2004), 8.

Chapter 5

1. Carl von Noorden, "Obesity," in his *Metabolism and Practical Medicine*, trans. I. Walker Hall (London: Heinemann Press, 1907), III: 693–715.

2. Noorden, "Obesity," 710.

3. Carl von Noorden, *Clinical Treatises on the Pathology and Therapy of Disorders of Metabolism and Nutrition. Obesity: The Indications for Reduction Cures*, trans. Boardman Reed (New York: E. B. Treat, 1903); here, 12.

4. Noorden, *Clinical Treatises*, 15.

5. Noorden, *Clinical Treatises*, 22.

6. Noorden, *Clinical Treatises*, 28.

7. Noorden, *Clinical Treatises*, 31.

8. Noorden, *Clinical Treatises*, 54.

9. Carl von Noorden, *Die Fettsucht* (Wien: Alfred Hölder, 1910), 63.

10. George Henry Lane Fox Pitt-Rivers, *The Clash of Culture and the Contact of Races* (London: Routledge, 1927), 82.

11. Robert Saundby, "Diabetes mellitus," in Thomas Clifford Allbutt, ed., *A System of Medicine* (London: Macmillan, 1897), 197–99.

12. Francis Howard Humphris, *Electro-Therapeutics for Practitioners* (London: Henry Frowde and Hodder & Stoughton, 1921), 206–19; here, 209.

13. W. S. Hedley, *Therapeutic Electricity and Practical Muscle Testing* (Philadelphia: P. Blakiston's Son and Co., 1900), 206–10.

14. Sigmund Freud, *Standard Edition of the Complete Psychological Works of Sigmund Freud*, ed. and trans. J. Strachey, A. Freud, A. Strachey, and A. Tyson, 24 vols. (London: Hogarth, 1955–74); here, 14: 9.

15. Lulu Hunt Peters, *Diet and Health, with Key to the Calories.* (Chicago: The Reilly and Lee Co., 1918), 12.

16. Peters, *Diet and Health*, 13.

17. Peters, *Diet and Health*, 16.

18. Frederick Gowland Hopkins, *Chemistry and Life.* Gluckstein Memorial Lecture 4 (London: Institute of Chemistry, 1933); here, 3.

19. Hopkins, *Chemistry and Life*, 5.

20. Hopkins, *Chemistry and Life*, 6.

21. William Withey Gull, *A Collection of the Published Writings of William Withey Gull*, 2 vols. (London: New Sydenham Society, 1896).

22. Hilde Bruch, *The Importance of Overweight* (New York: Norton, 1957), 5.

23. Bruch, *The Importance of Overweight*, 138.

24. Bruch, *The Importance of Overweight*, 140.

25. Hilde Bruch, "Gaswechseluntersuchungen über die Erholung nach Arbeit bei einigen gesunden und kranken Kindern" Dissertation (Freiburg im Breisgau, 1928), 10; simultaneously published in the *Jahrbuch für Kinderheilkunde*, 121 (1928), 7–28.

26. Sigmund Freud, "Psychical (or Mental) Treatment (1890)" in Freud, *Standard Edition of the Complete Psychological Works of Sigmund Freud*, ed. and trans. J. Strachey, A. Freud, A. Strachey, and A. Tyson, 24 vols. (London: Hogarth, 1955–74), I: 283–4.

27. Felix Deutsch, "Studies in Pathogenesis: Biological and Psychological Aspects," *Psychoanalytic Quarterly*, 2 (1933), 225–43; here, 235–6.

28. Franz Wittels, "Mona Lisa and Feminine Beauty: A Study in Bisexuality," *International Journal of Psycho-Analysis*, 15 (1934), 25–40; here, 28.

29. A. H. Vander. "Review of 'Hilde Bruch, Obesity in Childhood'," *Psychoanalytic Quarterly*, 13 (1944), 131.

30. A. H. Crisp and Edward Stonehill, "Treatment of Obesity with Special Reference to Seven Severely Obese Patients," *Journal of Psychosomatic Research*, 14 (September 1970), 327–45; here, 342.

31. Henry B. Richardson, "Obesity and Neurosis," *Psychiatric Quarterly*, 20 (1946), 400–4.

32. C. M. Louttit, *Clinical Psychology of Children's Behavior Problems* (N. Y. & London: Harper & Brothers, 1947), 639.

33. *Psychoanalytic Review*, 35 (1947), 103–5.

34. Gustav Bychowski, "On Neurotic Obesity," *Psychoanalytic Review*, 37 (1950), 301–19.

35. R. N. Aruffo, "Lactation as a Denial of Separation," *Psychoanalytic Quarterly*, 40 (1971), 100–22.

36. S. Aronson, "The Bereavement Process in Children of Parents with AIDS," *Psychoanalytic Study of the Child*, 51 (1996), 422–35.

37. J. R. Bemporad, E. Beresin, J. J. Ratey, G. O'Driscoll, K. Lindem, and D. B. Herzog, "A Psychoanalytic Study of Eating Disorders," *Journal of the American Academy of Psychoanalysis*, 20 (1992), 509–31.

38. Psyche A. Williams-Forson, *Building Houses out of Chicken Legs: Black Women, Food, and Power* (Chapel Hill, NC: University of North Carolina Press, 2006).

39. Daniel Patrick Moynihan, *The Negro Family: The Case for National Action* (Washington DC: Office of Policy Planning and Research United States Department of Labor, 1965), 150.

40. *Diagnostic and Statistical Manual of Mental Disorders.* 4th edn., text revision (IV-R) (Washington: American Psychiatric Association, 2000), 583.

41. William R. Miller, ed., *The Addictive Behaviours: Treatment of Alcoholism, Drug Abuse, Smoking and Obesity* (Oxford: Pergamon Press, 1980).

42. Jane Wardle, Susan Carnell, Claire MA Haworth, and Robert Plomin, "Evidence for a Strong Genetic Influence on Childhood Adiposity Despite the Force of the Obesogenic Environment," *American Journal of Clinic Nutrition*, 87 (2008), 398–404.

43. J. W. Butters and T. F. Cash, "Cognitive-behavioral Treatment of Women's Body Image Dissatisfaction," *Journal of Consulting and Clinical Psychology*, 55 (1987), 889–97.

44. Kathleene Derrig-Palumbo and Foojan Zeine, *Online Therapy* (New York: Norton, 2005).

45. Michael R. Lowe, K. M.-K., Nema Frye, and Susan Phelan, "An Initial Evaluation of a Commercial Weight Loss Program: Short-Term Effects on Weight, Eating Behaviours and Moods," *Obesity Research*, 7 (1999), 51–9.

46. G. Ken Goodrick, Kay T. Kimball, Rebecca S. Reeves, and John P. Foreyt, "Non-Dieting Versus Dieting Treatment for Overweight Binge-Eating Women," *Journal of Consulting and Clinical Psychology*, 66 (2) (1998), 363–8.

47. C. G. Fairburn, "Interpersonal Psychotherapy for Bulimia Nervosa," in D. M. Garner and P. E. Garfinkel, eds., *Handbook of Treatment for Eating Disorders* (New York: Guilford Press, 1997), 278–94.

48. Collen S. Rand and Albert J. Stunkard, "Psychoanalysis and Obesity," *Journal of the American Academy of Psychoanalysis*, 5 (1977), 459–97.

49. Colleen Heikel, Michell Rosenfeld, and Anees A. Sheikh, "Imagery in Smoking Cessation and Weight Management," in Anees A. Sheikh, ed., *Healing Images: The Role of Imagination in Health* (Amityville, NY: Baywood Publishing, 2003), 223–54.

50. D. L. Johnson and R. T. Karkut, "Participation in Multicomponent Hypnosis Treatment Programs for Women's Weight Loss With and Without Overt Aversion," *Psychological Reports*, 79 (1996), 659–68; here, 664.

51. M. A. Gravitz, "Early Uses of Hypnosis in Smoking Cessation and Dietary Management: A Historical Note," *American Journal of Clinical Hypnosis*, 31 (1988), 68–9.

Chapter 6

1. Jean Vague, "La différenciation sexuelle: facteur déterminant des formes de l'obesité," *Presse Médicale*, 30 (1947), 339–40.

2. Susie Orbach, *Fat is a Feminist Issue: How to Lose Weight Permanently Without Dieting* (New York: Paddington Press, 1978), 4.

3. Kim Chernin, *The Obsession: Reflections on the Tyranny of Slenderness* (New York: Harper and Row, 1981), 35.

4. Michael L. Power and Jay Schulkin, *The Evolution of Obesity* (Baltimore: The Johns Hopkins University Press, 2009), 41.

5. Virginia W. Chang and Nicholas A. Christakis, "Medical Modeling of Obesity: A Transition from Action to Experience in a Twentieth-century American Medical Textbook," *Sociology of Health and Illness*, 24 (2002), 151–77.

6. Power and Schulkin, *The Evolution of Obesity*, 41–2.

7. Yiying Zhang, Ricardo Proenca, Margherita Maffei, Marisa Barone, Lori Leopold, and Jeffrey M. Friedman, "Positional Cloning of the Mouse Obese Gene and its Human Homologue," *Nature*, 372 (1994), 425–31.

8. Zhang *et al.*, "Positional Cloning of the Mouse Obese Gene," 431.

9. J. M. Friedman, "A War on Obesity, Not the Obese," *Science*, 299 (2003), 856–8.

10. Leonard Williams, *Obesity* (London: Humphrey Milford, Oxford University Press, 1926), 53.

11. See Jean Leray, *Embonpoint et Obésité* (Paris: Masson et Cie, 1931), 11–12; W. F. Christie, *Surplus Fat and How to Reduce It* (London: William Heinemann, 1927), which begins with a long discussion of racial predisposition to fat, 1–8.

12. W. H. Sheldon, S. S. Stevens, and W. B. Tucker, *The Varieties of Human Physique* (New York: Harper & Brothers, 1940), 221.

13. Richard M. Goodman, *Genetic Disorders Among the Jewish People* (Baltimore: Johns Hopkins, 1979), 334–41; citing K. Schmidt-Nielsen, Howard B. Haines, and Donald B. Hackel, 'Diabetes Mellitus in the Sand Rat Induced by Standard Laboratory Diets', *Science* 143 (1964), 689.

14. Nikhil V. Dhurandhar, "Infectobesity: Obesity of Infectious Origin," *Journal of Nutrition*, 131 (2001), 2794S–7S.

15. Dhurandhar, "Infectobesity."

16. Deborah Jones, "Vaccine may Target Obesity in the Future," Agence France Presse, in English (October 18, 2005 Tuesday 4:36 p.m. GMT).

17. Marilynn Marchione, "Virus Is Linked To Weight Problems In Humans," *Seattle Post-Intelligencer*, (April 8, 1997).

18. M. J. Lyons, I. M. Faust, R. B. Hemmes, D. R. Buskirk, J. Hirsch, and J. B. Zabriskie, "A Virally Induced Obesity Syndrome in Mice," *Science*, 216 (1982), 82–5.

19. Kathleen Lebesco, *Revolting Bodies: The Struggle to Redefine Fat Identity* (Boston: University of Massachusetts Press, 2004), 112–3.

Chapter 7

1. "Preliminary Report of Committee on Infant and Invalid Diet," *China Medical Journal*, 26 (1912), 133–44.

2. Mary Stone, "Hospital Dietary in China," *China Medical Journal*, 26 (1912), 298–301; here, 299.

3. B. E. Read, "Some Factors Controlling the Food Supply in China," *China Medical Journal*, 25 (1921), 1–7.

4. Hartley Embrey and Tsou Ch'ing Wang, "Analysis of Some Chinese Foods," *China Medical Journal*, 35 (1921), 247–57.

5. W. H. Adolph and P. C. Kiang, "The Nutritive Value of Soy Bean Products," *China Medical Journal*, 34 (1920), 268–75; William H. Adolph, "Diet Studies in Shantung," *China Medical Journal*, 37 (1923), 1013–19.

6. Thus the journal regularly reprints summaries of Western medical essays, such as one taken from the *Berliner Klinische Wochenschrift* of March 1914 advocating "cream and bed rest": *China Medical Journal*, 29 (1915), 419–20.

7. Jean I. Dow, "Maternity Famine Relief," *China Medical Journal*, 36 (1922), 59–67.

8. Letter to the editor by Sargent, "The Trade in Chinese Children," *China Medical Journal*, 34 (1920), 695.

9. Thus, in an editorial, "Relation of Oriental Diet to Disease," *China Medical Journal*, 38 (1924), 834–36, the concern is about diseases ranging from appendicitis to gall stones to cancer.

10. Quoted in Vivienne Lo and Penelope Barrett, "Cooking Up Fine Remedies: On the Culinary Aesthetic in a Sixteenth-century *Materia Medica*," *Medical History* 49 (2005), 395–422; here, 417.

11. William Hamilton Jefferys and James L. Maxwell, *The Diseases of China: Including Formosa and Korea* (1911), 320.

12. Thomas King Chambers, "On The Pathology of Obesity," *Boston Medical and Surgical Journal*, 43 (1851), 9–16.

13. Thomas B. Futcher, "Diabetes Mellitus and Insipidus," in William Osler, ed. *Modern Medicine: Its Theory And Practice* (Philadelphia and New York: Lea & Febiger 1914), 1: 674–728; here, 1: 674–5.

14. Jefferys and Maxwell, *The Diseases of China*, 259.

15. James L. Watson, "Food as a Lens: The Past, Present, and Future of Family Life in China," in Jun Jing, ed., *Feeding China's Little Emperors: Food, Children, and Social Change* (Stanford University Press, 2000), 199–212; here, 208.

16. Wang Dungen, "Reforming the Human Body" ("*Renti Gailiang*"), *Shenbao Ziyoutan*, (August 29, 1911), 3.

17. Mao Zedong, "A Study of Physical Education" (April 1917), in *Mao's Road to Power: Revolutionary Writings 1912–1949*, ed., Stuart R. Schram, 5 vols. (Armonk, NY: M. E. Sharpe, 1992–99), vol. 1, (1992): 113–27.

18. Watson, "Food as a Lens", 208.

19. Shuhui and Weiseng, "On Obesity" ("Lun Feipang Zhi Bing"), *Funu Shibao* [*Women's Newspaper*], 10 (April 1913), 26–8.

20. Wilhelm Ebstein, *Die Fettleibigkeit (Corpulenz) und ihre Behandlung nach physiologischen Grundsätzen*, 6th edn. (Wiesbaden: J. F. Bergmann, 1884), 10.

21. Daizuo, "Keep the Body Slim" ("Jianshou Ja"), *Jiating Zizhi* [*Family Magazine*], 3 (1922), 1–4; here, 1.

22. W. S. Hedley, *Therapeutic Electricity and Practical Muscle Testing* (Philadelphia: P. Blakiston's Son and Co., 1900), 209–10.

23. Zhou Zhenyu, "The Cause and Danger of Female Obesity," ("Funu Feipang De Yuanyin He Haichu"), *Xin Nuxing* [*The New Woman*], 1 (1926), 42–5. Published in Shanghai, this journal had a reputation for its views on sexuality and health.

24. "What Causes Obesity?" *Journal of the American Medical Association*, (September 27, 1924), 1003.

25. Qihui, "Tragedy at the Dinner Table" ("Canzhuoshang De Beiju"), *Liangyou*, 167 (June 1941), unpaged.

26. Watson, "Food as a Lens", 208.

27. T. Colin Campbell and Junshi Chen, "Diet and Chronic Degenerative Diseases: A Summary of Results from an Ecological Study in Rural China," in Norman J. Temple and

Denis P. Burkitt, eds., *Western Diseases: their Dietary Prevention and Reversibility* (Totowa NJ: Humana Press, 1994), 67–118.

28. Longde Wang, Lingzhi Kong, Fan Wu, Yamin Bai, and Robert Burton, "Preventing Chronic Diseases in China," *The Lancet*, 366 (November 19–25, 2005), 1821–4; here, 1821; see also Dongfeng Gu, Kristi Reynolds, Xigui Wu, *et al.*, "Prevalence of the Metabolic Syndrome and Overweight Among Adults In China," *The Lancet*, 365 (April 16–22, 2005), 1398–1405.

29. G. S. Ma, Y. P. Li, Y. F. Wu, *et al.*, "[The Prevalence of Body Overweight and Obesity and Its Changes Among Chinese People during 1992 To 2002]," *Zhonghua Yu Fang Yi Xue Za Zhi* [*Chinese Journal of Preventive Medicine*], 39 (2005), 311–5.

30. Xiaoping Weng and Benjamin Caballero, *Obesity and Its Related Diseases in China: The Impact of the Nutrition Transition in Urban and Rural Adults* (Youngstown, NY: Cambria Press, 2007), 1.

31. W. P. Jia, K. S. Xiang, L. Chen, J. X. Lu, and Y. M. Wu, "Epidemiological Study on Obesity and its Comorbidities in Urban Chinese Older than 20 years of Age in Shanghai, China," *Obesity Reviews*, 3 (2002), 157–65.

32. Weng and Caballero, *Obesity and Its Related Diseases in China*, 17–18.

33. See James L. Watson, "China's Big Mac Attack," in James L. Watson and Melissa L. Caldwell, eds., *The Cultural Politics of Food and Eating: A Reader* (Oxford: Blackwell, 2005), 70–9.

34. James L. Watson, ed., *Golden Arches East: McDonald's in East Asia* (Stanford, CA: Stanford University Press, 2006), vii.

35. Watson, *Golden Arches East*, 186–7.

36. Watson and Calwell, *The Cultural Politics of Food and Eating*, 78.

37. Yunxiang Yan, "McDonald's in Beijing: The Localization of Americana," 39–76; here, 71; James L. Watson, ed., "McDonald's in Hong Kong: Consumerism, Dietary Change, and the Rise of a Children's Culture," in *Golden Arches East: McDonald's in East Asia* (Stanford, CA: Stanford University Press, 2006), 77–1009; here, 89–90.

38. David Y. H. Wu, "McDonald's in Taipei: Hamburgers, Betel Nuts, and National Identity," in James L. Watson, ed., *Golden Arches East: McDonald's in East Asia* (Stanford, CA: Stanford University Press, 2006), 110–35; here, 133.

39. Tsung O. Cheng, "Obesity in Chinese Children," *Journal of the Royal Society of Medicine*, 97 (May 2004), 254.

40. Zumin Shi, Nanna Lien, Bernadette Nirmal Kumar, Ingvild Dalen, and Gerd Holmboe-Ottesen, "The Sociodemographic Correlates of Nutritional Status of School Adolescents in Jiangsu Province," *Journal of Adolescent Health*, 37 (2005), 313–22.

41. J. X. Jiang, X. L. Xia, T. Greiner, G. L. Lian, and U. Rosenqvist, "A Two Year Family Based Behaviour Treatment for Obese Children," *Archives of Disease In Childhood*, 90 (2005), 1235–8.

42. B. Xie, C. P. Chou, D. Spruijt-Metz, *et al.*, "Effects of Perceived Peer Isolation and Social Support Availability on the Relationship between Body Mass Index and Depressive Symptoms," *International Journal of Obesity*, 29 (2005), 1137–43.

43. Neeraj Kaushal, *Do Food Stamps Cause Obesity? Evidence from Immigrant Experiences* (Cambridge MA: NBER, [January] 2007).

44. Jyu-Lin Chen and Christine Kennedy, "Factors Associated With Obesity in Chinese-American Children," *Pediatric Nursing*, 31 (2005), 110–15; here, 111. The American context is vital. It is very much different from the health worries of the Chinese Diaspora in today's urban Britain. See Ruby C. M. Chau and Sam W. K. Yu, "Pragmatism, Globalism and Culturalism: Health Pluralism of Chinese People in Britain," in Ian Shaw and Kaisa Kauppinen, eds., *Constructions of Health and Illness: European Perspectives* (Aldershot: Ashgate, 2004), 65–79.

45. Chen and Kennedy, "Factors Associated With Obesity in Chinese-American Children," 115.

46. G. G. Harrison, M. Kagawa-Singer, S. B. Foerster, H. Lee, *et al.*, "Seizing The Moment: California's Opportunity to Prevent Nutrition-Related Health Disparities in Low-Income Asian American Population," *Cancer*, 104 (2005), Suppl: 2962–8.

47. Michael McCarthy, "Stunted Children are at High Risk of Later Obesity," *Lancet*, 349 Issue 9044 (January 4, 1997), 34.

48. Weili Yan, Xiaoyan Yang, Yujian Zheng, *et al.*, "The Metabolic Syndrome in Uygur And Kazak Populations," *Diabetes Care* 28 (2005), 2554–5.

49. Frank Dikotter, *The Discourse of Race in Modern China* (Stanford, CA: Stanford University Press, 1992).

50. Jing Tsu, *Failure, Nationalism, And Literature: The Making of Modern Chinese Identity, 1895–1937* (Stanford: Stanford University Press, 2005).

51. Jean Eid, Henry G. Overman, Diego Puga, and Matthew A. Turner, *Fat City: Questioning the Relationship Between Urban Sprawl and Obesity* (London: CEPR, [March] 2007), 1.

52. W. P. T. James, "Appropriate Asian Body Mass Indices," *Obesity Reviews*, 3 (2002), 139. This is still being debated in 2005: Tsung O. Cheng, "Using WHO's Body Mass Index Cutoff Points to Classify as Overweight and Obese Underestimates the Prevalence of Overweight and Obese among the Chinese," *International Journal of Cardiology*, 103 (2005), 343.

53. Y. Tahara, K. Moji, S. Muraki, S. Honda, and K. Aoyagi, "Comparison of Body Size and Composition Between Young Adult Japanese-Americans and Japanese Nationals in the 1980s," *Annals of Human Biology*, 30 (2003), 392–401.

54. Naomi Moriyama, *Japanese Women Don't get Old or Fat: Secrets of My Mother's Tokyo Kitchen* (New York: Delacorte, 2005).

55. Moriyama, *Japanese Women don't get Old or Fat*, 8.

56. Moriyama, *Japanese Women don't get Old or Fat*, 25.

57. Theodore C. Bestor, "How Sushi Went Global," in James L. Watson and Melissa L. Caldwell, eds., *The Cultural Politics of Food and Eating: A Reader* (Oxford: Blackwell, 2005), 13–20.

58. Richard Parish, "Health Promotion: Rhetoric and Reality," in Robin Bunton, Sarah Nettleton and Roger Burrows, eds.,

Sociology of Health Promotion Critical Analyses of Consumption, Lifestyle and Risk (London: Routledge, 1995), 13–23.

59. T. Colin Campbell and Thomas M. Campbell II, *The China Study: The Most Comprehensive Study of Nutrition Ever Conducted and the Startling Implications for Diet, Weight Loss and Long-Term Health* (Dallas: Benbella Books, 2005), 69–110.

60. Campbell and Campbell II, *The China Study*, 75.

61. Weng and Caballero, *Obesity and Its Related Diseases in China*, xi.

62. G. Li, X. Chen, Y. Jang, *et al.*, "Obesity, Coronary Heart Disease Risk Factors and Diabetes in Chinese: An Approach to the Criteria of Obesity in the Chinese Population," *Obesity Reviews*, 3 (2002), 167–72; here, 167.

63. "Malnutrition Hits 30 Percent of China's Poverty-stricken Children: Survey," *Agence France Presse*, (October 8, 2005).

64. Clay Chandler, "Little Emperors: China's Only Children— More than 100 Million of Them—Make up the Largest Me Generation Ever. And Their Appetites are Big," *Fortune*, (October 4, 2004), 138–42.

65. Chandler, "Little Emperors."

66. D. G. Chen, X. F. Cheng, and L. L. Wang, "Clinical Analysis of 200 Cases of Child Anorexia," *Chinese Mental Health Journal* 7 (1993), 5–6; in Chinese.

67. Jun Jing, "Introduction," in Jun Jing, ed., *Feeding China's Little Emperors: Food, Children, and Social Change* (Stanford University Press, 2000), 1–26; here, 5.

68. Jing, "Introduction," 5.

69. Jing, "Introduction," 9.

70. L. S. Adair and B. M. Popkin, "Are Child Eating Patterns Being Transformed Globally?" *Obesity Research*, 13 (2005): 1281–99.

71. http://ific.org/foodinsight/2001/jf/globesityfi101.cfm.

72. Thus, a leaflet handed out outside McDonald's in Leicester Square, London in April 2004 criticized McDonald's as

exploiting workers, damaging the environment, farming animals under cruel conditions, and promoting food which "is linked with a greater risk of heart disease, cancer, diabetes and other diseases." *What's Wrong With McDonald's? Anti-McDonald's Campaign* (Nottingham: Anti-McDonald's Campaign, [2004]). Certainly the major book on this topic remains Eric Schlosser, *Fast Food Nation: The Dark Side of the All-American Meal* (New York: Perennial, 2002).

73. Yunxiang Yan, "Of Hamburger and Social Space: McDonald's in Beijing," in James L. Watson and Melissa L. Caldwell, eds., *The Cultural Politics of Food and Eating: A Reader* (Oxford: Blackwell, 2005), 80–103; here, 82.

74. Jun Jing, ed., *Feeding China's Little Emperors: Food, Children, and Social Change* (Stanford University Press, 2000), 213–17.

75. M. T. Cabioglu and N. Ergene, "Electroacupuncture Therapy For Weight Loss Reduces Serum Total Cholesterol, Triglycerides, and LDL Cholesterol Levels In Obese Women," *The American Journal of Chinese Medicine*, 33(2005): 525–33.

Chapter 8

1. Donna Eberwine, "Globesity: The Crisis of Growing Proportions," *Perspectives in Health*, 7 (3) (2002), 6–11; here, 8.

2. Jean Anthelme Brillat-Savarin, *The Physiology of Taste or, Meditations on Transcendental Gastronomy*, trans. M. F. K. Fisher (Washington: Counterpoint, 1999), 239 and 241.

3. Immanuel Kant, *Immanuel Kant's Menschenkunde. Nach handschriftlichen Vorlesungen*, ed. Friedrich Christian Starke (Leipzig: Die Expedition des europäischen Aufsehers, 1832), 299.

4. Christopher William Hufeland, *The Art of Prolonging Life*. 2 vols. (London: J. Bell, 1797), 169.

5. Edmund Gayton, *The Art of Longevity, or, A Diaeteticall Institution* (London: printed for the author, 1659), 25–6.

6. Georg Forster, *A Voyage Around the World*, 2 vols., ed. Nicolas Thomas and Oliver Berghof (Honolulu: University of Hawaii Press, 2000), 164–5.

7. James Cook, *A Voyage Towards the South Pole, and Round the World. Performed in His Majesty's Ships the Resolution and Adventure, in the Years 1772, 1773, 1774, and 1775* (London: printed for W. Strahan; and T. Cadell, 1777), 347.

8. Edwin James, *Early Western Travels, Vol. 15: Part II of James's Account of S. H. Long's Expedition, 1819–1820*, ed. Reuben Gold Thwaites (Cleveland: A.H. Clark Co., 1905), 68.

9. John B. Wyeth, *Early Western Travels, vol. 21: Wyeth's Oregon, or a Short History of a Long Journey, 1832: Townsend's Narrative of a Journey Across the Rocky Mountains, 1834*, ed. Reuben Gold Thwaites (Cleveland: A.H. Clark Co., 1905), 307.

10. "Scottish Peasantry," *The Weekly Entertainer* (London), 59 (1819), 672–4; here, 674.

11. Edmund Blunden, *Leigh Hunt's "Examiner" Examined* (London: Harper & Brothers, 1931), 23.

12. Chandler Robbins, *Remarks on the Disorders of Literary Men, or, An Inquiry into the Means of Preventing the Evils Usually Incident to Sedentary and Studious Habits* (Boston: Cummings, Hillard, 1825), 56–7.

13. Robbins, *Remarks on the Disorders of Literary Men*, 58.

14. Robbins, *Remarks on the Disorders of Literary Men*, 57.

15. William Newnham, *Essay on the Disorders Incident to Literary Men: And on the Best Means of Preserving Their Health, Read before The Royal Society of Literature, Nov. 5, 1834* (London: John Hatchard and Sons, 1836), 3.

16. Robbins, *Remarks on the Disorders of Literary Men*, 31–2.

17. Sander L. Gilman, "Black Bodies, White Bodies: Toward an Iconography of Female Sexuality," *Critical Inquiry*, 12 (1985), 203–42.

18. Frances Galton, *Narrative of an Explorer in Tropical South Africa* (1852; London: Ward, Lock and Co, 1890), 97.

19. Galton, *Narrative of an Explorer in Tropical South Africa*, 129.

20. Galton, *Narrative of an Explorer in Tropical South Africa*, 202.

21. Galton, *Narrative of an Explorer in Tropical South Africa*, 53–4.

22. William Mavor, *An Historical Account of the Most Celebrated Voyages, Travels, and Discoveries, From the Time of Columbus to the Present Period* (Philadelphia: Samuel F. Bradford, 1802), 18.

23. Thus, Aldo Castellani and Albert J. Chalmers, *Manual of Tropical Medicine*. 3rd edn. (London: Baillière, Tindal and Cox, 1919), do not reflect this as a problem at all.

24. Michael Gelfand, *The Sick African* (Cape Town: Stewart Printing, 1944); diseases of nutrition, 153–70; obesity, 306.

25. Cyril Percy Donnison, *Civilization and Disease* (Baillière & Co.: London, 1937).

26. Donnison, *Civilization and Disease*, vii.

27. Donnison, *Civilization and Disease*, 6.

28. Donnison, *Civilization and Disease*, 2.

29. Donnison, *Civilization and Disease*, 29.

30. Donnison, *Civilization and Disease*, 30.

31. Donnison, *Civilization and Disease*, 30.

32. Julian Huxley, *African View* (London: Chatto and Windus, 1931), 162.

33. Hugh Trowell, "Hypertension, Obesity, Diabetes mellitus and Coronary Heart Disease," in H. C. Trowell and D. P. Burkett, eds., *Western Diseases: Their Emergence and Prevention* (London: Edward Arnold, 1981), 3–32; here, 14.

34. Trowell, "Hypertension, Obesity..." 65.

35. Trowell, "Hypertension, Obesity..." 70.

36. Trowell, "Hypertension, Obesity..." 70.

37. Weston Price, *Nutrition and Physical Degeneration. A Comparison of Primitive and Modern Diets and Their Effects, etc.* (Redlands, CA: Published by the Author; New York, London: P. B. Hoeber, 1939), 5.

38. Price, *Nutrition and Physical Degeneration*, 353.

39. Price, *Nutrition and Physical Degeneration*, 498.

40. Price, *Nutrition and Physical Degeneration*, 43.

41. Price, *Nutrition and Physical Degeneration*, 509.

42. S. B. Eaton, Marjorie Shostak, and Melvin Konner, *The Paleolithic Prescription: A Program of Diet & Exercise and a Design for Living* (New York: Harper & Row. 1988).

FURTHER READING

Chapter 1

George A. Bray, "A Brief History of Obesity," in Christopher G. Fairburn and Kelly D. Brownell, eds., *Eating Disorders and Obesity: A Comprehensive Handbook* (New York: Guilford Press, 2002), 382–7.

Christopher E. Forth and Ana Carden-Coyne, eds., *Cultures of the Abdomen* (New York: Palgrave, 2005).

Michael Gard and Jan Wright, *The Obesity Epidemic: Science, Morality, and Ideology* (London; New York: Routledge, 2005).

Joyce Louise Huff, "Conspicuous Consumptions: Representations of Corpulence in the Nineteenth-century British Novel," Dissertation (George Washington University, 2000).

Heather McLannahan and Pete Clifton, eds., *Challenging Obesity: The Science Behind the Issues* (Oxford: Oxford University Press, 2008).

Lee F. Monaghan, *Men and the War on Obesity: A Sociological Study* (London: Routledge, 2008).

Gail Turley Houston, *Consuming Fictions: Gender, Class, and Hunger in Dickens' Novels* (Carbondale: Southern Illinois University Press, 1994).

Chapter 2

David Haslam and Fiona Haslam, *Fat, Gluttony and Sloth: Obesity in Medicine, Art and Literature* (Liverpool: Liverpool University Press, 2009).

Elena Levy-Navarro, *The Culture Of Obesity in Early and Late Modernity: Body Image In Shakespeare, Jonson, Middleton, and Skelton* (New York; Basingstoke: Palgrave Macmillan, 2008).

Chapter 3

Lucian Boia, *Forever Young: A Cultural History of Longevity from Antiquity to the Present* (London: Reaktion Books, 2004).

Anita Guerrini, *Obesity and Depression in the Enlightenment: The Life and Times of George Cheyne* (Norman: The University of Oklahoma Press, 2000).

Sidney W. Mintz, *Tasting Food, Tasting Freedom: Excursions into Eating, Culture, and the Past* (Boston: Beacon Press, 1996).

Chapter 4

Kerry Segrave, *Obesity in America, 1850–1939: A History of Social Attitudes and Treatment* (Jefferson, NC: McFarland & Co., 2008).

Peter N. Stearns, *Fat History: Bodies and Beauty in the Modern West* (New York: New York University Press, 1997).

Chapter 5

Jane Ogden, *The Psychology of Eating: From Healthy To Disordered Behavior* (Malden, MA: Blackwell, 2003).

Hillel Schwartz, *Never Satisfied: A Cultural History of Diets, Fantasies, and Fat* (New York: The Free Press, 1986).

Bill Lambrecht, *Dinner at the New Gene Café: How Genetic Engineering is Changing What We Eat, How We Live, and the Global Politics of Food* (New York: St. Martin's Press, 2001).

Chapter 6

A. H. Lichtenstein, "Dietary Fat: A History," *Nutrition Reviews*, 57 (1999), 11–14.

Samantha Murray, *The 'Fat' Female Body* (Basingstoke: Palgrave Macmillan, 2008).

Barry M. Popkin, *The World Is Fat: The Fads, Trends, Policies, and Products That Are Fattening The Human Race* (New York: Avery, 2009).

Ruth Raymond Thone, *Fat—A Fate Worse than Death: Women, Weight, and Appearance* (New York: The Haworth Press, 1997).

Chapter 7

T. Colin Campbell and Junshi Chen, "Diet and Chronic Degenerative Diseases: A Summary of Results from an Ecological Study in Rural China," in Norman J. Temple and Denis P. Burkitt, eds., *Western Diseases: Their Dietary Prevention and Reversibility* (Totowa NJ: Humana Press, 1994), 67–118.

H. T. Huang, *Science and Civilisation in China. Biology and biological technology. Fermentations and Food Science* (Cambridge: Cambridge University Press, 2000) vol. 6, part 5.

Frederick J. Simoons, *Food in China: A Cultural and Historical Inquiry* (Boca Raton: CRC Press, 1991).

Xiaoping Weng and Benjamin Caballero. *Obesity And Its Related Diseases In China: The Impact Of The Nutrition Transition In Urban And Rural Adults* (Youngstown, NY: Cambria Press, 2007).

Chapter 8

Francis Delpeuch, *Globesity: A Planet out of control?* (London, Sterling, VA: Earthscan, 2009).

Diana Wylie, "Disease, Diet, Gender: Late twentieth-century Perspectives on Empire," *Oxford History of the British Empire* (Oxford: Oxford University Press, 1999), vol. 5: 277–89.

INDEX

aboulia 59
Ad-36 virus 124, 125
addiction 115
    to food 107
adventitia 36
allopathic medicine 69, 130,
    166, 173
Americanization 144–5
    KFC 153, 154
    McDonald's 145–6
    Pizza Hut 154
android obesity 113
anorexia nervosa 94, 96, 106,
    111, 173
    ghrelin in 120
anti-obesity anxiety 138–9
appetite 42
appetite suppressants 31–2
Aristotle 24–5
Arnald of Villanova, *Salernitan
    Regime of Health* 35–6
Asia
    diet 150
    obesity in 149–50
Asian-Americans 147
athletic training 25
Atkinson, Richard 124
Atwater, Wilbur Olin 80
Augustine of Hippo 32–3,
    41–2
    City of God 33–4
Aulus Cornelius Celsus 25–6
Aytoun, William E. 66

bad genes 107–8
bad parenting 97, 102, 105–7
Banting, Frederick 85
Banting, William 61–6, 83
    *Letter on Corpulence Addressed
        to the Public* 61
bariatric surgery 123–4, 173
Battle Creek Sanitarium 67–8,
    70, 71, 74, 75, 76
Beard, George Miller 69
Beecher, Catharine 72
behavioral therapy 108
Benedict, Francis Gano 81
    *A Biometric Study of
        Basal Metabolism in
        Man* 81
    *An Experimental Inquiry
        Regarding the Nutritive Value
        of Alcohol* 81
Bergonié, Jean-Alban 87
Bernard, Claude 64, 80, 90
Best, Charles Herbert 85
Bin Xie 146
Blount, Thomas 60–1
body
    as God's temple 32
    ideal 34
Body by God Plan 77
body dysmorphic disorder 111
body image 108, 114
body mass index (BMI) 173–4
body weight monitoring 45
Bonaparte, Napoleon 19

Boswell, James, *The Life of Samuel Johnson* 61
Bouchardat, Apollinaire 95
Bowditch, Henry Pickering 89
Bradshaw, Watson 65
Bright, Edward 4
Brillat-Savarin, Jean Anthelme 64, 159–60
  The Physiology of Taste or, Meditations on Transcendental Gastronomy 59
Bruch, Hilde 94–100, 102–3, 106–7
  Eating Disorders 17–19, 96
Bruyère, Jean de La 46
bulimia 111
Burwell, C. Sidney 16–17
Butters, Jonathan 108
Bychowski, Gustav 104

Caelius Aurelianus 24
calorie counting 91
calories 174
Cannon, William Bradford 89–90
  Bodily Changes in Pain, Hunger, Fear, and Rage 90
  The Wisdom of the Body 90
Cash, Thomas, *Body-Image Therapy: A Program for Self-Directed Change* 109
Chen Duxiu 136
Chen, Jyu-Lin 146
Cheng, Tsung O. 145
Chernin, Kim 114, 128
Cheyne, George 52–6
  Essay on Health and Long Life 52
  The English Malady, or, a Treatise of Nervous Diseases of all Kinds, as Spleen, Vapours, Lowness of Spirits, Hypochondrical, and Hysterical Distempers 52

childhood obesity 4–20, 96–7
  and developmental disruption 102
  and poor parenting 97, 102
children, overindulgence of 47
China
  Americanization 144–5
  attitude to obesity 131
  child malnutrition 152–3
  diet 151
  fear of obesity 142–3
  "Little Emperors" 153–4
  minority groups 148
  New Woman (*xin nuxing*) 136
  obesity in 132–3, 134
  parenting style 146–7
  prevalence of obesity 143–4
  spread of McDonald's 145–6
  thinness as undesirable 136–7
  Westernization 131, 144–5, 151
  Westernized Modern Girl (*modeng nulang*) 136
Chinese medicine 130–57
  Hanshu 137
  "immoderate body" 133–4
  "new body" 135–6, 140–1
  obesity treatments 156–7
  Phragmites communis Trirn 137
Christianity, body as God's temple 32, 34
chymoi see humors
Constantine of Carthage 31
Cooke, Josiah Parsons 81
Cornaro, Alvise Luigi 38–44
  Discourses on a Sober Life 38
corpulence 36, 51–2, 65

Darwin, Charles 121
Davenport, Charles B. 89
degeneracy 159, 164–5
Deng Xiaoping 153
desire 10–11
Deutsch, Felix 100

Dhurandhar, Nikhil 124–5
diabetes 84–5
  as failure to adapt 123, 152
  as Jewish disease 86–7, 122
Dickens, Charles
  Fat Joe 4–15
  Mr Pickwick 5
  Pickwick Papers 4–15
diet 29
  balance in 47
  China 151
  definition of 59–60
  Japan 150
  natural 165
dieting 110, 164, 174
  first book on 31
  moral value of 56
  see-saw 55
diets, religion-based 77
Dionysus of Carystus 23
diseases of extravagance 159
diuretics 29
Don, W.G., Fat Boy 11–12
Donnison, Cyril Percy 166
dying well 39
dyspepsia 69

eating disorders
  anorexia nervosa 94, 96, 106,
    111, 120, 173
  bulimia 111
  therapy for 109–10
eating as healing (*diatetica*) 23
Ebstein, Wilhelm 7
Eddy, Mary Baker 75
electroacupuncture 156–7
electrotherapy 87–9
Elsholtz, Johann Sigismund,
  Diaeteticon 45
Enlightenment 38–57
Epicureans 33
Esquirol, J.E.D. 59
etiology 174

eugenics 86, 121
exercise, desirability of 25, 28,
  29

failure of mind 59, 94
Fairburn, Christopher 111
family unit, collapse of 106–7
famine 132, 142
fasting 57
fat
  bad qualities of 46
  giving meaning to 120–1
fat camps 131
Fat Joe 4–15
  attraction to Mary 10–11
  diagnoses of condition 15–16
  inscrutability of 7–8
  mental/emotional status 6–7
  narcolepsy of 13
Fat Liberation Manifesto 128
fat tax 127
Fat Underground 128
fatness
  excessive 24
  gender differences 23–4
  and longevity 24–5
  as sign of gluttony 34
fertility, obesity affecting 140
fitness culture 77
Flemyng, Malcolm, *A Discourse
  on the Nature, Causes, and
  Cures of Corpulency* 51
Fletcher, Horace 164
food
  addiction to 107
  correct preparation of 28–9
  desire for 33
  healthy 45–6, 150, 171
  "natural" 159
  temperature of 163–4
  unhealthy 45–6
food faddism 169
Ford, Henry 70

Forster, Georg 160–1
Franklin, Benjamin 49–50
Freud, Sigmund 89, 98–101
Friedman, Jeffrey 117
Froehlich's syndrome 15
Fromm-Reichmann,
    Frieda 96

Galen 27–8
  non-natural causes of
    illness 27–8
  On the Fat and Lean Mode of
    Life 28
  On the Nature of Foods 28
Galton, Francis 121–2, 164
gastric motility, studies on 90
Gelfand, Michael, *The Sick*
    African 166
gender differences 23–4
gender politics 84
genetic studies 116–20
genetics 174
ghrelin 120
Gilman, Charlotte Perkins, *The*
    Yellow Wallpaper 84–5
globalization 145, 174
globesity 20, 158–72, 174
gluttony 32, 38, 141
  forms of 34–5
goiter 171
Gompers, Samuel 77
Graham, Sylvester 72–3
  Lecture to Young Men on
    Chastity 73
  Lectures on the Science of Human
    Life 73
  Treatise on Bread, and
    Bread-Making 72
Grape-Nuts 76
Greek medicine 21–5
Griesinger, Wilhelm 94
Griffin, Ward 123
growth hormone 116

Gula 59
Gull, William 94, 95
gymnastics 25
gynoid obesity 113

Hallelujah Diet 77
Harris, James Arthur, *A*
    Biometric Study of Basal
    Metabolism in Man 81
Harvey, William 4, 64, 66
healthy foods 45–6
Herodicus of Selymbria 25
Himsworth, Harold
    Percival 122
Hippocrates 21–2, 24, 25
Hirsch, Jules 116, 126
Hoover, Herbert 91
Hopkins, Frederick
    Gowland 93
hormones 80, 116, 174–5
Hottentots, as "degenerates"
    164–6, 167
Hufeland, Christoph
    Wilhelm 160
  The Art of Prolonging Life 46
humors 21–3, 175
Huxley, Julian 168
hygiene 68
hypnotism 112
hypopituitarism 15
hypothyroidism 14–15

Ibn Sina, *Kitab al-Quanun* 31
idleness 47
ileum 175
immoderation 46
infantilism 99
infection 175
infectobesity 124, 126, 175
International Size Acceptance
    Association 128
Internet-driven interventions
    109–10

Isaac Judaeus 30–1
  Kitab al-adwiya al-mufrada wal-aghdhiya 31
Ito, Chikashi 123

James, Edwin 161
James, William 75, 89
Jameson, Thomas 51
Japanese food, health qualities of 150
Japanese paradox 150
jejunoileal bypass 123, 175
jejunum 175
Jews
  diabetes as Jewish disease 86–7, 122
  obese stereotype 86, 97, 122
  perceived healthiness of kosher food 171
Jiang, J.X. 146
Johnson, Samuel 60–1, 62
  views on obesity 61
Judaism 28–32
  attitude to obesity 30, 31–2
  dietary rules 29–30
Jukes, Edward 12
Jun Jing 154, 155

Kant, Immanuel 48, 160
  "Overcoming Unpleasant Sensations by mere Reasoning" 48–9
Kellogg, John Henry 67, 69–70, 71–2
  Plain Facts about Sexual Life 69
  'The San' 70–1
  The Stomach: Its Disorders and How to Cure Them 69
  Tobaccoism or How Tobacco Kills 69
Kellogg, William Keith 71, 76
Kellogg's Cornflakes 76
Kennedy, Christine 146

KFC 153, 154
kosher food, perceived healthiness of 171
Kuriyama, Shigehisa, *The Expressiveness of the Body and the Divergence of Greek and Chinese Medicine* 130

Lambert, Daniel 1–3
Leclerc, Georges-Louis 74
leptin 19, 117, 119
Li Shizhen, *Bencai gangmu* 133–4
libido theory 111
Lichtenberg, Georg 7
Lidz, Theodore 96
Liebig, Justus von 93
life expectancy 114
  moderation and long life 41–2
Louttit, C.M., *Clinical Psychology of Children's Behavior Problems* 104
lust 32–3

McDonald's 145
Maimonides, *Regimen of Health* 31
Maker's Diet 77
Mao Zedong 136, 142, 153
Mason, Edward 123
mastication 164
materialism 175
Maudsley, Henry, *Body and Mind: An Inquiry Into Their Connection and Mutual Influence* 59
mental imagery 112
Mercuriale, Gerolamo 36
Meredith, George 3
metabolic syndromes 144
Minadoi, Tommaso 36
Mitchell, S. Wier 84
moderation, and long life 41–2

molecular markers 118
Moore, A.W. 65
moral panic 106, 115–16, 175
Morgagni, Giovanni
     Battista 46
Morselli, Enrico 111
mouse studies 117
Moynihan, Patrick 107

narcolepsy 13
National Association to
     Advance Fat
     Acceptance 128
natural foods 159
"natural man" 162–3
   illness of 171
   Scots vs English 162
neurasthenia 176
Newnham, William 164
Niemeyer, Felix 67
"noble savage" 159–60
Noeggerath, Carl 97
Noorden, Carl von 82–6
nutrition, science of 93

ob-gene 117–18, 121, 123
obesitas 25, 36
obesity 176
   Asia vs West 149
   dangers of 138–9
   as disease 23, 26, 51, 62–3
   as failure of mind 59
   and fertility 140
   history of 21–37
   introduction as medical
      term 60–1
   as sin 32, 34–5, 38
   social stigma 63, 127
   types of 137
   ugliness of 138
   viral origin 124
obesity epidemic 115, 126, 142
obestatin 120

obsessive-compulsive
     disorder 107
obstructive sleep apnea 16–17
Oedipal conflict 104–5
old age
   decline in 49
   healthy 43–4
Orbach, Susie 113
Ord, William 14
Overeaters Anonymous 78
overeating 24

Paleolithic diet 171–2
parenting styles 146–7
Parrish, Richard 150
Paul of Aegina 29
Paul of Tarsus 33–4
Penney, J.C. 70
Perky, Henry 74–5
Peters, LuLu Hunt 91–3
   Dieting and Health, With Key to
      the Calories 91
phlegm, and predisposition to
     fat 23, 24
Phragmites communis Trirn 137
Pickwick Syndrome 16–17
Pierce, Deborah, I Prayed Myself
      Slim 77
Pitt-Rivers, George 86
Pizza Hut 154
plethos 28
polysarkia 24, 28
Post, Charles William 74–7
   death of 77
   I am Well! The Modern Practice of
      Natural Suggestion as Distinct
      from Hypnotic Unnatural
      Influence 75
   La Vita Inn 75
Pratt, E.H. 77
Price, Weston, Nutrition and
      Physical Degeneration 169
primitive races 168–9

psychoanalysis 17–18, 98,
    99–100
psychodynamic theory 104
psychological theory 94–5
psychopathology 100
ptomaine 69–70, 176
public weighing 45

Queen Victoria 19

Rabec, Claudio 19
Reid, Thomas 59
Renaissance period 38–57
Ribot, Théodule, *The Diseases of
    the Will* 59
Robbins, Chandler 163
Rockefeller, John D. 70
Rollo, John 85
Roman medicine 25–9
Röntgen, Wilhelm 90
Roosevelt, Franklin D. 19
Rousseau, Jean-Jacques 56
Roux-en-Y gastric by
    pass 123–4
rye, healthy qualities of 170

Sanctorius Sanctorius, *De statica
    medicine* 45
St Teresa of Avila 35
scholars 162–3
Schwendes, Valentin 31
see-saw dieting 55
self-abuse 68, 73
self-control, lack of 30
self-harm 105
Sen, Amartya, *Poverty and
    Famines: An Essay on
    Entitlement and
    Deprivation* 132
sexual reform 68
Shedd, Charlie, *Pray Your Weight
    Away* 77
Sheldon, W.H. 122

Sims, Ethan Allen 117
slow metabolisers 92–3
snack calories 155
sobriety 40
Social Darwinism 75
Socrates 24
somatic 176
Spencer, Herbert 3
stigmatization of obesity 63, 127
Stoics 33
sushi 150

Tahiti 161
talk-therapy 111
Tandler, Julius 82
temperance 41
Thevenot, Melchisedec, *The Art
    of Swimming and Advice for
    Bathing* 50
Thomas Aquinas 34–5
thrifty gene 115, 122, 152
Tidy, H. Letheby 15
Trowell, Hugh 168
Trundley, Johnnie (Fat Boy of
    Peckham) 13–14
"tyranny of slenderness" 114,
    128
Tyron, Thomas
    Poor Richard's Almanack 50
    *The Way to Health, Long Life and
        Happiness* 49

unhealthy foods 45–6

Vague, Jean 113
Vander, A.H. 102
vegetarianism 54, 70, 176
viral origin of obesity 124
Voit, Carl von 80

Wang Dungen 135
Washburn, Arthur
    Lawrence 90

Watson, James L. 136, 142, 145
Watson-Williams, E. 15–16
Weight Watchers 110
Wesley, John 56–7
Westernization 131, 144–5, 151
What would Jesus Eat Program 77
White, Andrew Dickson 58
White, Ellen G. 67–9
Wittels, Franz 101
women
    anti-obesity anxiety 138–9
    obesity as disease of 91–2,
        138, 162

obesity and fertility 140
    Oedipal conflict 104–5
Wood, William 61
Wundt, Wilhelm 89
Wyeth, John 162
Wyndham, William 50

X-rays 90

Zhou Zhenyu 139
Zumin Shi 145
Zuntz, Nathan 80